Advanced Praise for *Disease-Proof Your Child*

"Yesterday I saw a child wearing a T-shirt that said, 'If you love me, don't feed me junk food.' I was delighted to see this, but I also know how difficult it can be to feed our children well, particularly when the foods that are most convenient and the most heavily advertised are often the ones we should avoid. Joel Fuhrman's new book is a blessing, because it makes it so much easier. It is excellent, and full of clarity, wisdom, and guidance you can trust. It can indeed give you the power to shape your child's health destiny."
> —John Robbins, author of *Diet for a New America*
> and *The Food Revolution*

"Should be required reading for every parent."
> —Howard F. Lyman, author of
> *The Mad Cowboy* and *No More Bull!*

"Joel Fuhrman, M.D., shares his nutritional and healing wisdom in this practical, readable book. [It] will help you give your offspring the healthiest start possible."
> —Michael Klaper, M.D., director of the
> Institute of Nutrition Education and Research,
> Manhattan Beach, California

"Children don't need to be chronically sick—as children or adults. Dr. Fuhrman's book compels parents to rethink the way they raise their children, starting with what they eat."
> —James Craner, M.D., M.P.H., consultant in
> occupational and environmental medicine, Reno, Nevada,
> and assistant clinical professor in the
> Department of Medicine, University of California,
> San Francisco School of Medicine

"A powerful tool for insuring that the children you love will live healthy and happy lives."

—Doug Lisle, Ph.D., and Alan Goldhamer, D.C.,
authors of *The Pleasure Trip*

"Dr. Fuhrman's book offers your family the solution to the epidemic of obesity and sickness that afflicts nearly every child eating the rich Western diet."

—John McDougall, M.D., director of the
McDougall Live-in Program, Santa Rosa, California

"If you truly love your children and your grandchildren, or if you are simply concerned about the health of the nation, then read this book and put it into practice. It's light-years ahead and is a magnificent source of salvation for our children."

—Groesbeck P. Parham, M.D., professor of
gynecologic oncology and preventive medicine and
senior scientist at the Comprehensive Cancer Center,
University of Alabama at Birmingham

"The natural, clean, and simple approach to eating described in this book represents the ideal for healthy living today and preventing disease tomorrow. The connection between nutrition and disease is very real. There is abundant evidence that using the healthy food choices advocated for by Dr. Fuhrman will make a significant difference in the ability of children as well as adults to fight disease. If we as a society could even partially shift our approach to eating in the direction of the recommendations made in this book, we would see dramatic improvements in the challenges we currently face with obesity and many other childhood diseases."

—Wayne S. Dysinger, M.D., M.P.H., chairman of the
Department of Preventive Medicine,
Lorna Linda University

Disease-Proof
Your Child

Also by Joel Fuhrman, M.D.

Fasting and Eating for Health:
A Medical Doctor's Program for Conquering Disease

Eat to Live: The Revolutionary Formula for
Fast and Sustained Weight Loss

Disease-Proof Your Child

Feeding Kids Right

....

Joel Fuhrman, M.D.

ST. MARTIN'S PRESS NEW YORK

www.stmartins.com

Design by Level C

LIBRARY OF CONGRESS CATALOGING-IN-PUBLICATION DATA

Fuhrman, Joel.
    Disease-proof your child : feeding kids right / Joel Fuhrman.—1st U.S. ed.
      p. cm.
    Includes bibliographical references (p. 223).
    ISBN 0-312-33805-8
    EAN 978-0-312-33805-3
    1. Children—Nutrition. 2. Diet therapy for children. 3. Children—Health and hygiene. I. Title.

RJ206.F797 2005
613.2'083—dc22

                                   2005040707

First Edition: August 2005

10 9 8 7 6 5 4 3 2 1

To my four wonderful children, who have made fatherhood
the most joyous and valuable thing I do.

Talia

Jenna

Cara

Sean

....

Contents

···········

Foreword

I commend Dr. Joel Fuhrman for writing this book, *Disease-Proof Your Child*. In recent decades, much has been written on the relationship of diet and health or, more to the point, of diet and disease. Much of this literature has dealt with the so-called chronic degenerative diseases like the cardiovascular diseases, cancers, diabetes, and obesity. These are the diseases that primarily occur during adulthood and that command so much of our total health care costs.

But, in this rush to elaborate this information, far too little attention has been given to childhood nutrition and its large contribution to our adult health. It is for this reason, among others, that I believe readers will find Dr. Fuhrman's book to be so valuable. For children, the diseases of concern to many are of the communicable and infectious types. Do the foods that protect against adult diseases like heart disease and cancer, for example, protect against childhood diseases as well—especially those like colds, flu, sore throats, and earaches that seem to come from school? Read this book and you will find plenty of evidence that the answer is a resounding yes. Healthy eating is a family thing: what is good for the young is also good for the elderly; what is good for one disease is mostly good for all diseases.

Dr. Fuhrman is well qualified to write this book—from several vantage points. As a doctor, he has had experience utilizing nutritional methods to help children in his practice; as an author, he brings credibility because of the standard of excellence in his highly successful book, *Eat to Live: The Revolutionary Formula for Fast and Sustained Weight Loss;* as a student of biomedical science, he is careful to reference his observations; and as a father of four children of his own, he knows what is possible.

Children are our future and it just makes common sense that the food they become accustomed to will likely be the food that they prefer for the rest of their lives. In today's society most children consume foods that will produce serious adult onset diseases down the road, and they do not eat the foods that may offer dramatic protection. But common sense doesn't always ring true for many people; they want empirical evidence, the scientific stuff. So, Dr. Fuhrman provides that evidence from the scientific literature and from his own practice.

In his practice, the good doctor's primary approach is to "do no harm," as the Hippocratic Oath dictates, and whenever possible he does this by choosing dietary change before choosing the nearest bottle of pills. His successes are impressive, not only because of his patient reports but also because these successes are substantiated in science. Nutritional science applied to the next generation can gift them a long and healthy life.

For those parents who are beholden to getting a prescription for their children's virus-induced colds and sore throats and earaches, a dietary remedy may come as a surprise. Making simple changes in the child's diet and lifestyle often can do more than pills and do it more safely. A good diet often solves both the immediate illness and, even more important, keeps future illnesses at bay.

Eating the right foods has far-reaching benefits, one of which means much less dependence on drugs. Remember that old adage: "an apple a day keeps the doctor away"? Dr. Fuhrman is making the same point—in his case, with lots of evidence. The excessive use of antibiotics is a good example. These drugs are being substantially oversubscribed, about ten times too much. Sadly, too many people still seem not to know that antibiotics don't work on viral diseases. This often does nothing for the illness but only leads to the development of antibiotic-resistant organisms that can cause a more serious problem in the future. Dr. Fuhrman also presents evidence that excessive use of antibiotics can lead to more problems, such as an increased risk of asthma and allergies.

Dr. Fuhrman's recommendations are simple yet profound. "Eat the right foods," he says, and "avoid physicians, medications and remedies" as much as possible.

Many will say that getting children to eat the right foods like vegetables, fruits, nuts, seeds, and whole grain products is very difficult if not impossible. I do not deny the difficulty, but it is here that Dr. Fuhrman's insight and advice shines. I agree with his conclusions and have also observed that both parents must really believe the advice they give their children and must eat the same foods. Our five grandchildren (7–13 years) have done well with their peers and willingly and proudly defend what they eat; so do the Fuhrman children. Healthy food can be almost addictive.

This is a book that should be on every physician's desk as well as in any home where there are children. Do it right and you will be surprised at the results. Your children deserve the best start in life possible.

T. Colin Campbell, Ph.D.,
author of *The China Study* and
Jacob Gould Schurman
Professor Emeritus of Nutritional Biochemistry
at Cornell University

....

Note to the Reader

The information in this book is provided to describe the dramatic health benefits of nutritional excellence started early in life. However, any decision involving the treatment of an illness should be made only after consulting the physician of your choice. Neither this nor any other book can guarantee complete absence of disease nor substitute for professional medical care or treatment. The names of patients discussed in this book have been changed, along with certain identifying characteristics.

....

Acknowledgments

I first have to acknowledge my wife, Lisa, for many reasons that I cannot list here. Not only does she put up with my arduous work and travel schedule, frequently being left alone to care for our four children, but she also supplies unflinching encouragement and sacrifice for my projects to reach fruition. She works as my partner to meet the needs of our family, business, and literary endeavors.

Many close friends of mine have assisted me with the book, notably Steven Acocella, D.C., and Barbara Sarter, Ph.D., who have helped me collect research; Marion Fanock, who has helped me with testing and modifying recipes; and Bob Phillips, who has assisted me in making charts and graphs.

I also acknowledge the many young people who allowed me to use their success stories in the book. Their names have been modified.

I am grateful to my literary agent, Mary Ann Naples, for all her out-of-the-ordinary contributions to this book and my work in general, and to the intelligent editing job by Sheila Oakes of St. Martin's Press. I also want to thank Marian Lizzi of St. Martin's Press for her enthusiastic support of this project.

....

We Are Molded by Our Childhood

When our son Elliot was three we already had a sickly child. He was suffering from his seventh ear infection this year and had severe eczema since his first year of life. We had been to numerous specialists for his raw, itchy skin and tried many medical treatments to no avail. My search for a better solution led me to Dr. Fuhrman. In only two months after changing Elliot's diet his skin condition has disappeared. To our surprise he never suffered another ear infection. It is not merely Elliot's recovery that has moved us to write, it is our enthusiasm and gratitude for the knowledge we have gained from Dr. Fuhrman that has given us an incredible sense of freedom and control over our own and our children's health.

—Leslie and Stuart Raymond

As parents, we want what is best for our children. We would never intentionally harm them—in fact, we make sure to get them the best possible care, read to them, play with them, and ensure their safety at home, at school, and at play. But when it comes to feeding them, somehow we don't know what's best. Our kids seem finicky and eat nothing but cheese or pasta or chicken fingers or milk and cookies, and we let them. At the same time, we notice that they are frequently ill—they suffer from recurring ear infections, runny noses, stomachaches, and headaches. We take them to the doctor, who prescribes yet another round of antibiotics. We assume, because we also see it happening with friends and family, that it is par for the course when bringing up children. It doesn't have to be so.

This scenario may be "normal" for kids today, but it is not normal for humans or any other species of animal that eats nutrient-rich natural foods. Scientific research has demonstrated that humans have a powerful immune system, even stronger than that of other animals, that makes our body a self-repairing, self-defending organism with the innate ability to defend itself against microbes and prevent chronic illness. The system operates at its best only if we give it the correct raw materials to work with. When a young body doesn't receive its nutritional requirements, bizarre diseases occur. Of late, there has been an increase in cancers that were unheard of in prior human history. Most of these can be linked to improper nutrition.

Despite our very best intentions, today there are health risks that well-meaning parents inflict on their children *without being aware of it.* Every day in small ways, we may well be causing harm to their precious little bodies through the choices we make about what we decide to feed them.

There is an issue of vital importance that most well-meaning parents are not aware of: *the modern diet that most children are eating today creates a fertile cellular environment for cancer to emerge at a later age.* Trying to prevent breast, prostate, and other cancers as an adult may not be totally possible because most risk factors cannot be changed at this late stage. The bottom line is that in order to have a major impact on preventing cancer we must intervene much earlier, even as early as the first ten years of life. In other words, *childhood diets create adult cancers.* When our children eat junk food instead of fruits and vegetables, the groundwork is being laid for cancer and other diseases to occur down the road.

Additionally, *many children today are very often recurrently sick with ear infections and allergies and then, later in life, may develop autoimmune illnesses such as lupus, ulcerative colitis, and rheumatoid arthritis.* The major contributor to the development of these illnesses is suboptimal nutrition. Kids become ill not *because they just naturally pass around germs or have bad genes, but because their diets are inadequate.* Medications cannot prevent these problems—only a diet of nutritional excellence can.

The most recent scientific evidence is both overwhelming and shocking—what we feed (or don't feed) our children as they grow from birth to early adulthood has a greater total contributory effect on the dietary contribution to cancers than dietary intake over the next fifty years. American children and most children in developed countries eat less than 2 percent of their diet from natural plant foods such as fruits and vegetables.[1] American children move into adulthood eating 90 percent of their caloric intake from dairy products, white flour, sugar, and oil. Amazingly, about 25 percent of toddlers between ages one and two eat no fruits and vegetables at all. By fifteen months, french fries are the most common vegetable consumed in America!

Childhood diets are unhealthy, but the issue goes beyond simple nutrition. Recent, compelling, scientific evidence over the past two decades has shown links between precise dietary factors and autoimmune illnesses such as Crohn's disease and lupus, as well as later-life cancers. This means that we now know what helps to create an environment in our bodies that is favorable for cancers to emerge later in life, and we understand how what they eat now can prevent cancer in our children's future. While the scientific evidence is in, parents haven't been informed that what their children eat during their growth years has such a profound effect on their later health and that the first ten years may be the most critical. Unfortunately, many parents are unwittingly feeding their children dangerous, cancer-provoking diets. My goal is to inform parents so that they can give their children the greatest gift of all: the opportunity for a long and healthy life.

This book reviews the scientific evidence and explains that *the vast majority of adult cancers are avoidable* if an excellent diet is begun and maintained from early childhood. Unfortunately, pediatricians and family physicians rarely discuss diet with parents, encouraging the perception that what a child eats does not matter. Parents also are uninformed that following an anti-cancer diet can free their children from repeated trips to the doctor, endless courses of antibiotics, and the curtailed living that comes from being frequently sick.

While the scientific information may be alarming, the solutions are simple. Eating to prevent common illnesses as well as to prevent life-threatening illnesses in the future can be easy and taste good. You and your family will discover that the right foods can protect against obesity, autoimmune disease, diabetes, heart disease, and cancer. It is my mission and my passion to get this vital information out to all parents, and I am not going to sugarcoat the message. The truth is too important. This book will show you the science and the solution—and you won't believe how easy and tasty it can be.

MY ROLES AS A PHYSICIAN AND A PARENT ARE SIMILAR

I have been a family physician for more than fifteen years. I chose the specialty of family practice because I knew the health of each family member is cohesively linked. I realized that in order to have a major impact on one family member, I had to affect the lifestyle and diet of the entire family unit.

I envisioned seeing everyone in the family and getting to know them all as their doctor and friend and becoming an extension of the immediate family, like in the old days, when everyone in town knew the doctor and paid him in home-grown produce and apple pie. I may not have received the bounty of the family farm, but I have been given the opportunity to care for and help many, many individuals and families. The results have been richly rewarding.

Most families seek me out because they are tired of having a perpetually sick child and have learned of my successes in helping children reclaim their health and stay well. The most common complaint is recurrent ear infections, and at the first visit many parents bring in a list of ten to twenty antibiotic prescriptions given to their child over the last year by their well-meaning family physician or pediatrician. Some of these children are faced with the prospect of undergoing sinus surgery or having tubes placed in their ears. Others are on drugs such as Ritalin for behavioral disorders. Doctors and parents tend to assume that because almost all children suffer from these common problems and frequent infections, they are normal.

When children are repeatedly or chronically ill, today's doctors treat patients as they were taught to—with antibiotics and other drugs. I see things very differently. If a child is repetitively or chronically ill, with one infection after another, I see that there is a problem with immunity—a problem that likely comes from an inadequate diet. I know that rather than antibiotics and other drugs, nutritional excellence must be the first choice in recovery and prevention. I have seen it work in my own practice. After seeing me and making dietary adjustments, almost every chronically ill child recovered and is able to maintain good health without resorting to more drugs and antibiotics.

I tell parents that if they follow my advice their child will no longer require frequent visits to the doctor. With most frequently ill children, more medical care or medicine is not the answer. Constant and frequent trips to the doctor actually illustrate a serious failure of the physician-patient and physician-family relationship.

A doctor who is concerned about his patient community is not merely concerned with solving an acute crisis that may arise, but also considers it time well spent to teach prevention. I have found, and the medical literature supports what I have seen in my practice, that true prevention includes superior nutrition. Remember, over 80 percent of all Americans die from cardiovascular disease, diabetes, and cancer, which are all diseases of nutritional ignorance.

More and more evidence emerges each year that the diets we eat in our childhood have far-reaching effects on our adult health and specifically on whether we get cancer. Similarly, there is an abundance of scientific research that supports the need for a dietary lifestyle that protects our children from other serious chronic diseases.

A REAL SOLUTION FOR PARENTS

Every day a parent asks, "When is your pediatric nutrition book coming out?" Parents are eager for information. They don't know what to feed their kids. They know that the diet of their household and of their community are unhealthy, but they don't know what to do. They are stumped because they want to make changes, but they don't know how to get their kids to like healthy foods. This book has the answers. Not only will it explain what a healthy diet is, it will show you how to implement the best diet for your children in such a way that they will love it, eat it, and adopt a healthy approach to nutrition that will last a lifetime.

As the father of three daughters and a son, I live the trials and tribulations of bringing up healthy children in our deeply unhealthy world. From bringing candy and doughnuts to soccer games to bringing cupcakes and ice cream to the classroom, many parents are unknowingly contributing to the ill health of their and others' children.

Although I don't expect every family to change their eating practices, I know that this book will forever change the way you look at what you are feeding your children.

American children are the heaviest worldwide, and they are getting heavier at a faster rate than other children around the globe.[2] This spread of obesity foreshadows an explosion in degenerative diseases such as diabetes, heart disease, and cancer waiting to erupt in our children's future. Together we can stop this tragedy from ever happening.

KIDS LOVE HEALTHY FOOD—HEALTHY FOOD LOVES THEM BACK

Because people have a tendency to be comforted by foods they were fed in childhood, changing to a healthful diet can take a good deal of effort. However, time and time again adults report that they like the healthful foods and anti-cancer diet as much as their prior one; it just takes time to adjust. The younger you are, the easier the adjustment. Children naturally love natural foods. Their genetic makeup is designed to consume nature's bounty without any coaxing or effort; they naturally like fruits and vegetables.

Not only do children like to eat healthy, but once they do they will reject junk food on their own. My medical practice over the last thirteen years has proved to me that children are willing and able to change dangerous habits more readily than adults. When I talk to elementary school students, they are invariably enthusiastic about eating healthy and learning about great-tasting healthy recipes. They often ask me how to get their parents to eat healthier or how their mom can learn to cook with healthy ingredients. In the presence of good information, they are hungry for knowledge, especially as it applies to their health. In elementary school, they readily learn the dangers of cigarette smoking and drugs. Likewise, they can easily learn the most important points about nutrition. If educated in a loving way, they enjoy eating healthy food and are proud of caring properly for their own bodies. My four children are a good example.

When Cara was four years old she brought defrosted, frozen broccoli spears, raw carrots, fruit, and raisins to preschool. Her friends' cookies, chips, and pretzels did not tempt her. She would brag, "I am never sick, because I eat healthy." Cara was never sick; she had no ear infections, no runny nose, and besides chicken pox, I only remember one viral illness her first seven years of life.

When Cara was seven years old, I picked her up from her morning summer camp at the local health club. The other kids were eating the snacks their parents had packed for them—chips, cookies, and candy, the usual stuff. We both noticed that all the other children were eating junk food. She asked me, "Don't these parents love their children?"

I said, "Of course they do, Cara; these parents just don't know that what they are giving their children will have such a harmful effect on their future health and happiness. That is one of my jobs in the future, to help these people learn how they can disease-proof their children, and maybe you can help me, too." Much of the idea and motivation to write this book was born in these important discussions with Cara and my other children.

Kids are not stupid; they grasp the simple concept that you are what you eat. Cara is ten now, but by the age of five she had more common sense about brushing her teeth and caring properly for her body than most adults I know.

Children understand that a loving parent makes sure they wear a seat belt, brush their teeth, and eat a healthy diet. Children understand that parents establish these habits and behaviors as an expression of love and that to do otherwise would potentially not only show a lack of caring, but damage their future health.

My middle daughter, Jenna, a thirteen-year-old, loves helping me figure out how to make healthy food designed for children's taste. I asked her, "How can we get kids to eat walnuts because they contain so many healthful compounds, including those important omega-3 fats?" She helped me design the Apple Walnut Surprise (see page 204.) That same night all my children ate it for dessert. Jenna loves having her friends who come over to the house help her make healthy recipes. Her favorite is her peach smoothie. She combines frozen or fresh peaches, soy milk, dates, and flax seeds and blends up a delicious yet healthful snack drink. Her friends love it, too. I thank Jenna for designing many of the recipes in this book and testing them on her friends. She is proud of her contribution to helping me get kids to eat healthy.

EATING HABITS TO LAST A LIFETIME

My four children eat green vegetables every day, even my three-year-old son, Sean. They have been fed them since infancy. By the time they were each five years old they knew lots of information about green vegetables. They learned that green vegetables are essential to create our body's immune system shield against dangerous diseases and lead to a healthy life span. They know that green vegetables have more nutrients per calorie than any other food and that at dinner every night we have a salad and a steamed green vegetable. They all like salads and greens and often snack on both raw and steamed string beans or steamed artichokes that sit on our kitchen island as they pass through the kitchen. Children learn the most from what their parents and the rest of the family do or don't do.

When a family moves to America from Thailand, they still shop for and eat Thai food. People have a tendency to like best what they are used to. Childhood eating habits established by the age of ten years old usually last a lifetime.

My daughter Jenna did not like chopped kale at first, but when she saw all of us eating it regularly and talking about how healthy it was, she tried it a few times. Interestingly, it has now become her favorite green vegetable. We like it best with the cashew cream sauce, a mix of raw cashews, soy milk, onion powder, and dehydrated vegetable seasoning.

My oldest daughter, Talia, who is in high school, is an example to both kids and parents who think that if you feed your children too healthfully when they are young, they will rebel and have an unhealthy relationship with food as they get older. On the contrary, she is not forced to eat healthy, she chooses to. She was raised in a loving environment where healthy foods, not unhealthy foods, were present. She also received a substantial education in nutrition as she grew up, so she knows the impact that food has on one's future health and well-being.

Talia is sensible. She does not eat perfectly all the time, but probably sticks with a healthy plant-based diet for all but a few meals per month. She has also learned that her friends do not want to be preached to or taught about food. She does not proselytize about the way she eats, but merely sets an excellent example for those around her. Without her trying to influence them, because of her example, her friends have started to eat healthier lunches, make better food choices, and ask her questions about her diet.

Combining what I know as a physician and what I've learned as a parent, this book brings you up-to-date medical and scientific information along with practical advice on how to use the best of that information in your own home. **Chapter 1** reviews a large body of nutritional information that explains the main problem with today's dietary practices and the key factors that are necessary to make your child disease-resistant. **Chapter 2** presents the basis of superior nutrition and applies it not merely to preventing illnesses, but gives clear guidelines to follow when your children are ill or faced with a health challenge. It also describes problems with conventional medical care and how the misuse and overuse of prescription drugs can harm our children. **Chapter 3** explains the causes of cancer and autoimmune illness and gives the scientific explanation of why most adult cancer is caused primarily by what we eat in our childhood. **Chapter 4** covers the problems people have with feeding their children and gives solutions to childhood feeding difficulties. It explains how to deal with the picky eater and exactly how to make the transition to optimal nutrition with your family. **Chapter 5** is your new family cookbook. It gives you the healthy meal plans and easy-to-make, kid-tested recipes that children love.

Being a father to my four children is the most meaningful and pleasurable part of my life. Our children are our most important and loved part of our world. Giving them the potential for a happy and healthy life is one of our greatest gifts to them.

Disease-Proof
Your Child

....

Understanding
Superior Nutrition

In order to better understand how our human bodies are programmed to process nutrients, we need to take a look at our closest wild relatives. Based on genetic information, gorilla and human DNA only differ by 1.8 percent. Chimpanzees are a little closer to humans, as their DNA differs by only 1.6 percent. Both humans and the larger primates share many physical and social characteristics: different body size for males and females, living in family groups, and mothers caring for offspring for a long time beyond infancy. Chimpanzees are dependent on their mothers until the age of seven. Primates are also very intelligent.

All primates (including humans) share certain nutritional requirements to maintain normal function and maintain excellent health. All primates can taste sweet and see color, and share a requirement for large amounts of antioxidants, phytochemicals, and other plant-derived nutrients such as vitamin C, vitamin K, and folate. The appreciation of sweets and the color vision attract us to and enable us to recognize ripe, fresh fruits, an important component of the natural diet of all primates. This desire of primates for variety in their diet supports nutrient diversity, enabling primates to live a long, disease-free life. Without an adequate amount of plant-derived nutrients, immune system dysfunction develops. This reduced function of the immune system occurs as a result of nutritional inadequacies, which may then result in frequent infections, allergies, and, eventually, cancer. Primates share this high requirement for natural foods found in nature's cupboard, the garden or the forest. The micronutrients that fuel the primate's immune system—derived from fruits and vegetables, nuts, seeds, beans, and, to a lesser degree, whole grains—must form the basis of the diet in order to expect normal resistance against disease.

Veterinarians and other animal-care workers are aware that for each species of animal to thrive they must eat a diet of natural foods that is uniquely suited to the nature of the species in question.

Humans suffer greatly from misunderstanding what our nutritional requirements are. We have evolved to a level of economic sophistication that allows us to eat ourselves to death. A diet centered on milk, cheese, pasta, bread, and sugar-filled snacks and drinks lays the groundwork for cancer, heart disease, diabetes, and autoimmune illnesses to develop later in life. It is not merely that sugar, other sweets, white flour, cheese, and butter are harmful; it is also what we are *not* eating that is causing the problem.

When you calculate all the calories consumed from the typical foods most children in America eat, you find that the calories coming from natural foods such as fresh fruit, vegetables, beans, raw nuts, and seeds is less than 5 percent of their total caloric intake. This dangerously low intake of unrefined plant foods guarantees weakened immunity to disease, frequent illnesses, and a shorter lifespan.

UNPROCESSED FOODS ARE THE KEY
TO OPTIMAL HEALTH

There are thousands of plant-derived nutrients that are essential for us to achieve proper functioning of our immune system. Let's look at just a few of these as an example.

Folate is found in vegetables, beans, and fruit. It is especially high in green vegetables. It was determined that the low level of folate in the modern American diet is related to an increased risk of neural tube defects in the womb. More recently, low levels of folate in the diet have been associated with other diseases as well, such as heart disease and breast cancer.[1] It is very likely that it is not lack of folate alone that is the chief player creating this increased risk, but also the lack of many other nutrients contained in folate-rich foods. Because the American diet is so low in fruits and vegetables, medical authorities advise women of childbearing age to take folate supplements. Instead of health authorities advising women of the dangers of a diet low in folate-rich green vegetables, they instead advise folate supplementation, as if dangerously low folate levels are the only problem with our nutritionally barren diet. Thousands of other health-supporting compounds would be ingested if women received their folate from greens, not pills. Typical nutritional advice, which focuses on individual nutrients instead of whole food, perpetuates the diet style that leads to serious illnesses.

Vitamin K is also found in green vegetables. It was found that low levels of vitamin K in mothers and their newborns increases the chance that the newborn will have a brain hemorrhage soon after childbirth. Because the American diet is low in vitamin K, all children born in hospitals in America are given a vitamin K shot immediately after delivery. Again, authorities offer fragmented nutritional advice instead of placing our respect in nature's nutrient sources, whole foods. Instead of advising mothers to eat more vegetables, and receive a symphony of valuable nutrients along with the vitamin K, we resort to giving all infants a vitamin K shot.

If women were instead educated about the critical importance of eating green vegetables and fresh fruit, instead of the present-day approach of encouraging folate supplementation and then giving all babies a vitamin K shot, possibly thousands of children would have been spared the tragedy of childhood cancers, from the improved dietary habits of pregnant women. Acute lymphoblastic leukemia (ALL) is the most common childhood cancer and, after accidents, is the most common cause of death in children. The low consumption of vegetables and fruits right before and during pregnancy has been implicated in its causation.[2]

As humans we have certain requirements for vitamins and minerals, and scientists have discovered many of these essential micronutrients and what role they play in the body. However, rather than eating whole foods and getting these nutrients in their natural state, we most often resort to supplements. Indeed, a billion-dollar nutritional supplement industry has erupted to the point where most Americans take many different nutritional supplements in an attempt to improve their health and prevent the development of diseases. However, this has not worked too effectively; those taking vitamin supplements are not granted protection from heart disease and cancer.

The problem with this fractionated way of thinking, simply replacing one nutrient or another through supplementation, is that there is much more than merely vitamin K and folate and a handful of other vitamins and minerals that are missed by not eating the required amount of fruits and vegetables.

Clearly, the modern American diet is inadequate, and in spite of most Americans taking nutritional supplements, the percentage of our population dying from the diseases of poor nutrition has not changed significantly in the last thirty years. Heart disease, diabetes, strokes, and cancer still kill more than 80 percent of all Americans. These same diseases kill those who take nutritional supplements and those who don't. We must look at the reasons why our society, so knowledgeable about vitamins and minerals, still suffers from such a high rate of diseases related to our diet.

Eating exceptionally healthfully is the foundation of our good health. Nutritional supplements add to the diet, and are not intended to take the place of healthy eating. That is why they are appropriately called *supplements*. A multivitamin is still a good idea for most people, and deficiencies of these commonly known nutrients do lead to higher risks of cancer. About forty vitamins and minerals are known to be required in the human diet. Deficiencies of vitamins B12 and B6, folic acid, niacin, iron, zinc, and selenium appear to mimic radiation damage by causing single- and double-strain breaks to our DNA.[3] Half of our population is deficient in vitamins and minerals, and these chronic low levels of nutrients lead to higher toxic elements within cells. The accumulation of these toxic by-products of metabolism accelerates cellular aging and creates an environment favorable for cancer to flourish. Low nutrient intake is a factor in the development of cancer and heart disease. Taking supplements, which supply various nutrients, may help somewhat, but it is not a sufficient solution. There is more to the cancer story.

In recent years, scientists have discovered another class of micronutrients, now called phytochemicals, that also play an indispensable role in enabling our normal defenses against cancer. The wave of new research on more than 12,000 recently identified phytochemical nutrients in natural (unprocessed) plant foods has generated excitement in the scientific community unparalleled since the first vitamin was discovered in the early 1900s. These nutrients work synergistically to detoxify cancer-causing compounds, deactivate free radicals, and enable DNA-repair mechanisms. These 12,000 or so phytochemicals play a major role in human immune system defenses. Without sufficient amounts and a wide variety of this new class of compounds, scientists noted, cells age more rapidly and do not retain their innate ability to remove and detoxify waste products and toxic compounds. This new class of antioxidant nutrients is essential to prevent the development of degenerative diseases. We cannot acquire a sufficient amount and diversity of phytochemicals in supplements; we must get them from real food, especially because many of them have not been discovered yet. When we pass up eating fruits and vegetables, we are turning our backs on a host of nutrients that can keep us from developing disease.

THE FOUNTAIN OF YOUTH

What we eat creates the materials to build our cells. Eventually, we are what we eat. When we eat certain foods we will achieve a body that nature designed to be disease-resistant; when we don't or when we eat the wrong foods, we may create a body that is disease-prone. The foods we eat supply us with much more than fuel. They provide the raw materials that make up our organs, including the brain. Critical nutrients make neurotransmitters and brain-cell receptors that govern how we think. Our diet supplies us with the raw materials to manufacture every cell comprising our body. These cells, to function at a high level, need thousands of different chemical compounds that combine in an amazing fashion to make the most miraculous machine ever created. When a few of these necessary compounds are missing, we usually can still survive; the human organism is resilient and adaptable, but without all the necessary components the body loses its powerful potential for wellness. As a result, chronic diseases develop.

Eating right won't simply prevent disease; it will help you live life to its fullest. Eating right will enable you to feel great every day, without stomachaches, headaches, indigestion, constipation, or a runny nose. The right nutrition can assure that we wake up fully energized and have boundless energy, perform at our best, and maintain our youthful vigor as we age gracefully. Eating healthfully can maintain your excellent health for a lifetime.

Health is normal. The human body is a self-repairing, self-defending, and self-healing marvel. Disease is relatively difficult to induce, considering the body's powerful immune system. However, this complicated and delicate machinery can be damaged if fed the wrong fuel during the formative years. The chronic diseases commonly associated with aging—hypertension, coronary artery disease, Type II diabetes, degenerative joint disease, Parkinson's, and Alzheimer's, as well as most cancers—are not the inevitable outcome of the aging process; they are born out of wrong food choices earlier in life.

Healthy living with nutritional excellence throughout life can slow the decline of aging. It can prevent the years and years of suffering in ill health that is so common today as people get older and become dependent on medical treatments, drugs, and surgery. Medical intervention does very little to slow the progression of illnesses and gradual mental and physical decline. Nutritional excellence is the only real fountain of youth.

VITAMINS AND MINERALS ARE NOT ENOUGH

Modern societies live mostly on processed foods. These foods have been developed to meet the requirements of mass production, shelf life, economics, and taste acceptance. These "fake foods" no longer resemble in any way the nutritional characteristics of real food made by nature. No matter how many vitamins or minerals are added to the power bar or breakfast cereal, it still does not contain the unique combination of thousands of delicate phytonutrients found in a strawberry or leaf of lettuce.

Natural foods deteriorate rapidly, have limited shelf life, and lose many of their delicate nutrients when heated, milled, or shot out of cannons. For example, cold breakfast cereals (which may have some synthetic nutrients that were lost in processing put back in) have as much phytochemical nutritional value as the cardboard box they are found in. We have adopted an eating pattern of the worst sort, consuming the majority of our caloric intake from processed foods, which pays us back with medical problems, unnecessary suffering, and a premature death.

Though many think that disease is the result of genetics or bad fortune, the reality is that for the vast majority, we will get what we have earned. Our body is formed from the foods we have consumed in our life. A body made from refined foods, white flour, oils, sugar, and other highly processed "fake" food develops into a sickly human, with allergies and autoimmune diseases, such as colitis, psoriasis, lupus, and asthma, who suffers from indigestion, reflux, headaches, irritable bowel syndrome, fibroids, tumors, and fatigue in early adulthood. Serious diseases that interfere with one's quality of life are born out of our childhood diets. Junk food isn't cheap; we pay a steep price for it years after consuming it.

THE GENETIC COMPONENT OF DISEASE

While genetics play a role in the expression of many diseases, and while we all have genetic weaknesses and predispositions, for the vast majority of diseases that occur in the modern world, nutrition, exercise, and environment play a much larger role than genetics. For example, those living in rural China have less than 2 percent heart disease risk, but when they move to America their children have the same dismal risks as other Americans. About 50 percent of Americans die of heart attacks and strokes. When we abuse our bodies, many different problems arise and what happens to you then may be influenced by your genetics.

Heart disease is a recent phenomenon in the history of mankind.[4] By 1916 it was already hypothesized by the well-known French scientist C. D. de Langen that overeating and a cholesterol-rich diet appeared to be a factor in the populations of those European countries experiencing a rise in heart attacks. We cannot consider heart disease to be primarily genetic, because it did not occur much before the last hundred years and pockets of populations inhabiting the world today have no heart disease. By the 1950s scientific investigations were able to explain population differences in heart disease rates by differences in the consumption of saturated fat (the most important determinant of serum cholesterol) and the inverse association with consumption of fresh produce.[5] The less saturated fat and the more fresh produce consumed, the less heart disease occurs. Over the last fifty years, this causal relationship between saturated fat and heart disease has been observed and documented by thousands of scientific studies. The reality is that heart disease, the leading cause of death in the modern world, as well as the other leading causes of death (various cancers and strokes), is created by our modern diet. Very few people have genetics so favorable that they can eat anything without concern.

You cannot escape from the biological law of cause and effect. Food choices, especially food choices early in life, are the primary cause of disease and premature death. Health predictably results from healthy living. Inferior childhood nutrition has led to a nation with high levels of chronic illnesses and out-of-control health care costs.

WHAT AMERICANS EAT

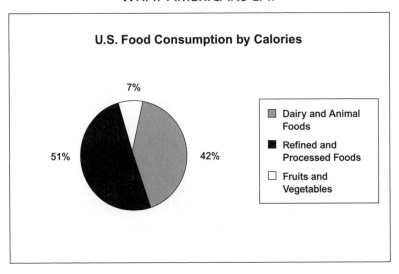

Americans eat about 40 percent of calories from animal products, such as meat, eggs, and dairy.

Animal products contain no antioxidants, bioflavonoids, carotenoids, folate, vitamin C, vitamin K, or those thousands of phytochemicals that are essential for cellular normalcy and preventing DNA damage.

Americans eat about 50 percent of calories from processed foods such as oil, sugar, and white flour products.

Processed foods contain almost no antioxidants, bioflavonoids, carotenoids, folate, vitamin C, vitamin K, or those thousands of phytochemicals that are essential for cellular normalcy and preventing DNA damage.

To make matters worse, most of the animal products eaten by children, such as cheese and milk, are exceptionally high in saturated fat. Saturated fat consumption correlates with cancer incidence worldwide.[6] It also raises cholesterol levels and causes heart disease.[7]

Keep in mind that it is the type of fat, not the amount of fat, that is linked to higher heart attack rates and cancer. Both epidemiologic studies and clinical trials have implicated saturated fats and trans fats as the villains for humans.[8] They promote both heart attack and cancer.

The nutrition committee of the American Heart Association has declared, ***There is overwhelming evidence that reduction in saturated fat, dietary cholesterol and weight offer the most effective dietary strategies for reducing total cholesterol, LDL levels and cardiovascular risk. There is no biological requirement for saturated fat.***[9]

In fact, populations with diets with little or no saturated fat have little or no heart disease. The development of heart disease begins in childhood. Not only do unhealthy childhood diets high in saturated fat and low in the protective micronutrients found in unpro-

Animal Fat Intake vs. Heart Disease

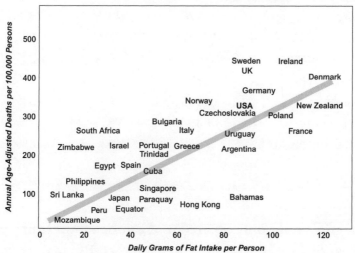

cessed plant foods accelerate heart disease, but they promote the aging process, and create a cellular environment favorable for the development of cancer.

To add insult to injury, much of the processed foods children eat are rich in trans fat, a man-made fat that is also linked to cancer and heart disease.[10, 11]

We could not have designed a cancer-causing environment more effectively if we scientifically planned it. We feed our children a diet high in saturated fat, add lots of processed foods with those dangerous (man-made) trans fats, and combine it with an insufficient intake of unrefined plant foods to guarantee sufficient phytochemical deprivation, and presto, we have created a nation rich in autoimmune illnesses, allergies, obesity, diabetes, and, finally, heart disease and cancer.

MAJOR FOODS: U.S. PER CAPITA FOOD SUPPLY—1996

	Weight in Pounds	Percentage by Weight	Percentage by Calories
Meats	192	8%	12%
Eggs	236	9%	7%
Dairy	576	23%	23%
Fruits and vegetables	**543**	**22%**	**5%**
White potatoes	153	6%	2%
Refined oils	67	3%	11%
Sweeteners	153	6%	13%
White flour	198	8%	9%
Other processed foods	378	15%	18%

Source: USDA Agriculture Fact Book 98: Chapter 1-A

Americans eat only 5 percent of calories from fruits, vegetables, beans, and unprocessed nuts and seeds, the foods that contain the necessary nutrients to maintain normal health.

Unless our diet is designed so our caloric consumption largely comes from these protective foods, we should not be surprised if our twenty-five-year-old daughter develops lupus or our eighteen-year-old son develops ulcerative colitis. Once they pass their child-bearing years, many of our children will be overweight; age rapidly; require drugs for hypertension, diabetes, and heart disease; have a heart attack; or die prematurely from cancer.

This can be avoided.

Cancer and heart disease have similar causes. Cancer kills about 35 percent of all adult Americans, heart disease and stroke about 50 percent. The more years of nutritional abuse and the earlier in life the abuse begins, the higher the risk.

Fatty Facts

- Saturated fat has the most powerful causative relationship with heart disease and cancer.

- Besides sugar, butter and cheese contribute the most calories to children's diets in America.

- The food with the highest saturated fat content in the American diet is butter and cheese.

Cheese consumption has tripled in America in the last thirty years, and cheese is included as a part of almost every meal. It's melted on burgers and chicken breasts, sprinkled on salads, melted over bread and pasta. It's not surprising that cheese gives us more (artery-clogging) saturated fat than any other food.

Heart disease begins in our youth and is not easy to reverse. No one should eat more than five grams of saturated fat a day. Over this level, disease rates climb.

All foods derived from animals contain cholesterol and tend

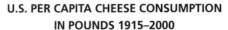

**U.S. PER CAPITA CHEESE CONSUMPTION
IN POUNDS 1915–2000**

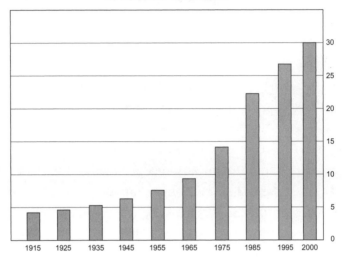

to be high in the thick, heavy fats called saturated fats. Most plant foods are very low in saturated fat, except for some tropical plant oils like palm and coconut oil that are naturally saturated.

Reducing the consumption of animal foods reduces the consumption of cholesterol and saturated fat. Low intake of cholesterol and saturated fat leads to a leaner body, clean arteries, and a reduced risk of developing heart disease and many other diet-related diseases such as stroke, breast cancer, colon cancer, diabetes, and obesity.

SATURATED FAT CONTENT OF COMMON FOODS[12]

	Grams of Saturated Fat
Cheddar cheese (4 oz)	24
American processed cheese (4 oz)	24
Ricotta cheese (1 cup)	20
Swiss cheese (4 oz)	20

Chocolate candy—semisweet (4 oz)	20
Cheeseburger, large, double patty	18
T-bone steak (6 oz)	18
Braised lamb (6 oz)	16
Pork—shoulder (6 oz)	14.5
Butter (2 tbsp)	14
Mozzarella, part skim (4 oz)	12
Ricotta cheese, part skim (1 cup)	12
Beef—ground, lean (6 oz)	11
Ice cream, vanilla (1 cup)	10
Chicken fillet sandwich	9
Chicken thigh, no skin (6 oz)	5
Whole milk, 3.3% fat (1 cup)	5
Plain yogurt	5
Two eggs	4
Chicken breast (6 oz)	3
Salmon (6 oz)	3
Walnuts 2 oz (24 halves)	3
2% milk (1 cup)	3
Tuna (6 oz)	2.6
Turkey, white, no skin (6 oz)	2
Almonds 2 oz (48 nuts)	2
Sunflower seeds (2 oz)	2
Flounder (6 oz)	0.6
Sole (6 oz)	0.6
Fruits	negligible
Vegetables	negligible
Beans/legumes	negligible

THE TRANS FAT NIGHTMARE

Many vegetable oils have been artificially saturated, or "hydro-genated," as the process is called. These "trans" fats are commonly used in processed junk foods such as candy bars, doughnuts, french fries, and snack foods.

Trans fat (also called phantom fat) is created during the process called partial hydrogenation, which involves turning liquid vegetable oils into solid shortening. Partially hydrogenated oils are used to make a wide variety of foods, including some cookies and snacks. Although some of these foods claim to be low in calories, fat, or cholesterol, the numbers are not listed for trans fat, which is even worse than cholesterol.

Trans fats are listed on boxes, wrappers, and jars as partially hydrogenated oil. This man-made food has been found to be as powerful as saturated fat in promoting disease. This problem is even more insidious because food manufacturers are not required to list the quantity of trans fat in their products.

Both saturated fat and trans fat raise the amount of LDL or bad cholesterol, but trans fat also lowers the amount of HDL or good cholesterol. The effect of saturated fat and trans fat on cholesterol levels is worse than the effect of eating cholesterol itself.

Fast food is typically very high in trans fat. French fries and other foods fried in partially hydrogenated oils are the worst. Also, be aware of any food fried in vegetable oil, too, because heating, cooling, and reheating oils causes chemical changes that create the negative effects similar to trans fat.

If you eat out in most restaurants and eat fast food, you are participating in high-risk behavior. Do not eat fried food. The only way to protect yourself is to eat wholesome food prepared at home or, if eating out, make sure you know what you are eating and how the dish was prepared.

SAMPLE FOODS LOADED WITH (DANGEROUS) TRANS FAT[13]

	Trans Fat Grams per 100 Grams Food
Margarine—stick	20
Corn oil or soybean oil spreads	17.6
Vegetable shortening	17
Potato chips	10.6
Margarine—tub	10
Chocolate chip cookies	9
Standard crackers	8.4
Taco shells	8
Microwaved popcorn (packaged)	7.7
Milk chocolate–coated cookie bar	6.9
Popcorn—oil-popped	6
French fries—fast food	5.2

Not only do processed foods and fast foods often contain dangerous trans fats and other additives, but they also can have high levels of acrylamides. When processed foods are baked and fried at high temperatures, these cancer-causing chemical compounds are produced. Many processed foods, such as chips, french fries, and sugar-coated breakfast cereals, are rich in acrylamides. Acrlyamides also form in foods you bake until brown or fry at home; they do not form in foods that are steamed or boiled.

There was worldwide alarm in the scientific community in 2002 after researchers announced that many of the foods children eat contain high levels of these potent cancer-causing compounds. Acrylamides cause genetic mutations, leading to a wide variety of cancers in lab animals, including breast and uterine cancer. It has not been definitively shown that acrylamides are a major factor in the development of human cancers, but most cancer experts working in this field presume that it does.[14] This offers another reason to avoid consumption of overly heated and processed foods.

NUTS, THE HIGH-FAT HEALTH FOOD

Many people, believing that fat is the culprit behind obesity, cancer, and heart disease, eat skinless chicken, fat-free mayo, and pasta. Unfortunately, a diet style centered on low-fat grains and lower-fat animal products is too low in the phytochemical-rich vegetation needed for adequate health. These people are also missing out on an adequate intake of minerals and healthy fats. The type of fat and the source of the fat are critical.

Raw nuts, seeds, and avocados are also foods rich in fat, but they contain healthy fats, important for normal growth and development, and they are rich in nutrients as well. Consumption of these foods has been shown to have powerful protective effects against disease. The results are so striking that in one study men who ate raw nuts had half the heart attack rate compared to men who did not eat nuts.[15] Furthermore, eating raw nuts and seeds has been shown to decrease the death rate from all causes, extending lifespan, and this effect was noted in various population groups, including whites, African Americans, and the elderly.[16] Eating nuts and seeds makes us live a lot longer and prevents both heart disease and cancer. Eating walnuts, almonds, pistachio nuts, sunflower seeds, flax seeds, and many more varieties is the best way for us, and especially our children, to get the healthy fats we need from nature's tasty and unpolluted source.

Humans and other primates are nut-eating mammals by design. These foods should be moved to a prominent place on our nation's food guide pyramid. Unfortunately, government-sponsored pyramids are strongly affected by social and political preferences; they do not directly reflect the scientific literature. When children obtain most of their essential fats from raw nuts and seeds, they not only get the healthier fats, but they also receive lots of beneficial minerals and antioxidants in the process.

Allergies to peanuts (which is actually a legume), which affect approximately 1 percent of children, have increased radically in developed countries, and allergy to tree nuts, though much less prevalent, has also increased. Research has demonstrated factors contributing to this recent skyrocketing of allergies including the use (misuse) of antibiotics early in life, brief or lack of breast-feeding, a too-early introduction of solid food, and the roasting of nuts.[17]

NUTRITION AND THE BRAIN

Mom's good nutrition during her pregnancy, the quality of her breast milk, and the foods children eat supply the raw materials to construct their brain and ultimately supply their brainpower. Nutrition in these critical early years of life is essential for each child to reach their maximum intellectual potential. Throughout life, what a person eats effects the levels of neurotransmitters and structure of cells and regulates all mental processes that affect how well we think and feel.

Scientists have noted that children who were breast-fed past the first birthday have better IQ scores than those raised on formula.[18] It was first thought that this was because breast milk, and (until very recently) not formula, contains omega-3 fatty acids and DHA, which are essential for optimal brain development. (Of course, the omega-3 content of breast milk is dependent on the mother's consumption of foods containing omega 3-fatty acids.) But more recently, science is discovering that many more nutrients can affect brain development besides DHA fat, and the mother's consumption of green vegetables and other produce can increase the nutritional content and diversity of nutrients in her breast milk. It is not surprising that an inadequate intake of any one of the forty-plus essential nutrients during the critical first few years of life has profound and lifelong effects on cognition memory and intelligence.[19] A complete symphony of phytonutrients in fruits, vegetables, beans, and nuts can be transmitted to the breast milk and play a role in healthy development of your child. Not only did researchers find breast-fed babies to be generally smarter than bottle-fed babies, but breast-fed babies from mothers who ate a very healthy diet (with lots of vegetables) throughout their pregnancy and nursing period gave their children the greatest capacity for brainpower later in life.

For many years, scientists believed that most brain development occurred in the first few years of life. However, it has been discovered that brain development continues well into the teenage years and beyond, meaning that optimal nutrition is critical over many years for maximum intelligence to be realized. Humans take so much longer to mature than other animals because our brain is so complicated and powerful that it takes a long time for this biologically advanced organ to finish developing.

Intelligence is influenced by nutritious eating. Only by maximizing nutritional factors favoring normal brain development can we maximize our intelligence potential. The same diet style that protects against aging and cancer helps our children increase their intelligence potential and protect their emotional well-being. Hyperactivity, attention deficit, depression, and other psychiatric disorders have their roots in early-life nutrition. The brain requires adequate nutrition to be a properly working machine. At younger ages the brain is most sensitive to negative nutritional influences.[20]

YOU BEHAVE AND THINK WHAT YOU EAT!

The brain is mostly made of fat. For the brain cells to maintain their cell membrane fluidity and to properly recognize chemical messengers they must have the right ratio of omega-6 and omega-3 fats built into their structure. Too little omega-3 fats and too much saturated fat and trans fat could stiffen the fatty acid membranes and interfere with proper cellular communication.[21] Raw nuts and seeds supply children with unpolluted omega-3 and omega-6 fatty acids in a protective package rich in antioxidant vitamins and minerals. Though fish is a rich source of omega-3 fat and DHA, fish fats and other animal fats are nutrient-poor and often contaminated with pollution, pesticides, hormones, and drugs. Flax seeds, sunflower seeds, sesame seeds, and walnuts are examples of great brain food that can maximize human potential. Berries and vegetables are also rich in brain-favorable nutrients. The same foods that provide powerful protective effects against cancer maximize our children's brain development.

When our children don't consume the right mix of brain-boosting nutrients, they have a reduced ability to learn and a lower IQ, and later in life they can develop dementia and Alzheimer's disease. On the other hand, the right mixture of brain-supporting foods will afford our children the ability to reach their maximum potential in life, not just for health, but for emotional stability, happiness, and success in their chosen careers.

OVERWEIGHT CHILDREN—GROWING IN THE WRONG DIRECTION

Obesity is the most common nutritional problem among children in the United States. One in three kids in America are overweight, and the problem is growing. The number of children who are overweight has more than doubled during the past decade. Social forces, from the demise of home cooking to the rise of fast food, as well as dramatic increases in snack food and soda consumption, have led to the most overweight population of children in human history. Added to this dietary disaster is television, computer, and video technology that entertains our youngsters while they are physically inactive. Unless parents take a proactive role in promoting and assuring adequate nutrition and an active lifestyle, you can be sure the children of America will continue this downward spiral into obesity and ill health. Obese children suffer physically and emotionally throughout childhood and then invariably suffer with adult heart disease, diabetes, and a high cancer incidence down the road.

Many schools and children's hospitals feature not only soda and snack machines but on-site outlets for fast-food chains. On a typical day, nearly one-third of American children ages four to nineteen are consuming fast food, according to a study of 6,212 children. Those children who ate fast food were found to have consumed more total fat, more added sugars, more sugar-sweetened beverages, less fiber, and fewer fruits and vegetables than those children who did not eat fast food. The children who ate fast food were also found to have consumed 187 additional calories a day, which could mean an extra six pounds per year per child.[22]

Children learn what to eat at their parents' table, and adults are eating more fast food, more convenience foods, and more unhealthfully than ever before in human history. Overweight parents don't just pass on the genes for obesity, but their eating habits as well. However, like every health condition, while genetics does play a role, it's not the major role.[23] It is what is put in front of our children for them to eat and drink that is the primary cause of childhood obesity.

Obesity rates have risen in tandem with soda consumption in the United States, and in the last twenty years the consumption of soft drinks by teenagers had doubled.[24] Twelve- to nineteen-year-old boys consume thirty-four teaspoons of sugar a day in their diet, and about half of that comes from soft drinks. Children start drinking soft drinks at a very young age, and advertisements and promotions by the soft drink manufacturers are aggressively marketed to the young.

ANNUAL SOFT DRINK PRODUCTION
IN THE UNITED STATES
(12-ounce cans per person)

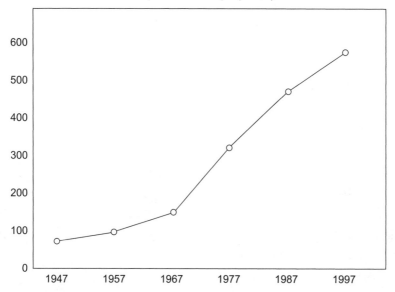

Source: Data from the National Soft Drink Association, Beverage World, *published by the Center for Science in the Public Interest (www.cspinet.org)*

Soft drinks and processed foods are full of high-fructose corn syrup (HFCS). HFCS is not only fattening, but this inexpensive and ultraconcentrated sugar has no resemblance to real food made by nature. It is another experiment thrust upon our unsuspecting children with unknown dangerous consequences. Besides sugar, corn syrup, and chemicals, these drinks often contain caffeine, an addictive stimulant. Children crave more and more as they get older. By adolescence most children have become soft-drink addicts. It is no surprise that six out of the seven most popular soft drinks contain caffeine. Contrast this high level of sugary "liquid candy" with the meager intake of fresh produce by children and teenagers, and it is no surprise that we have an obesity epidemic beyond all expectations.

CAFFEINE CONTENT IN COMMON SOFT DRINKS (mg/12 oz)

Coca-Cola	34
Diet Coke	46
Dr Pepper	41
Mello Yellow	53
Mountain Dew	55
Pepsi-Cola	38
Pepsi Diet	36
Tab	47

Source: National Soft Drink Association

Clearly, the major cause of this recent phenomenon of obesity is the availability and consumption of high-caloric, low-nutrient foods and the deceased consumption of high-nutrient foods. When families finally realize that the consumption of vegetables, beans, and fruits is the essential foundation of an adequate diet, we will rarely see an obese child. It is literally impossible to become obese when consuming a diet that predominates in healthful, natural food.

Our children need to be more physically active and exercise with sports and games, but with "fake food" so readily available, exercise alone will not solve the problem.

We cannot rely on the food manufacturer, our government, the media, or even health authorities to protect or warn us against the dangerous foods we feed to our children. Regardless of the political, economic, and social causes for the unhealthy meals served in our school cafeterias, parents bringing doughnuts to our children's schoolrooms, soda machines in our school cafeterias, and fast food franchises in our hospital lobbies, it is still our primary responsibility as parents to nurture, protect, and teach our children how to live, eat, and act sensibly in a world of dangerous opportunities. We all must accept the fact that health is created and experienced as a result of the healthful behaviors and environment we create for ourselves and our loved ones. We must take personal responsibility by educating ourselves and teaching our children to care for themselves.

Changing the way your child eats at home is the first place to lay the groundwork for a more healthful life. Children can readily pick up the bad habits that surround them, but you have the opportunity to teach them healthier eating habits that will last a lifetime and give them a longer, healthier life to boot.

SALTING AWAY OUR CHILDREN'S FUTURE— HYPERTENSION AND STROKES

Today, not only are the waists of children in America growing bigger and bigger, but the blood pressure of children has been steadily climbing over the last fifteen years.[25] Small increases in blood pressure in childhood predict big increases down the road.

A large body of data illustrates that populations with low salt consumption have lower levels of blood pressure compared to populations with higher salt intake. In Japan and China, salt intakes are often as high as eighteen grams or more per day. Hypertension (high blood pressure) and stroke are the major causes of premature death in these nations. The National Center for Health Statistics reports that in the United States, the mean salt intake is eight grams per day. This high intake of sodium assures that we have an elderly population with high blood pressure.

High salt intake, and resultant high blood pressure later in life, does not merely increase the risk and incidence of stroke. It also can lead to kidney failure, congestive heart failure, and heart attack. Raising our children on low-salt diets can have a major role in securing the future health of our nation. Salt intake also correlates with incidence of stomach cancer.[26]

Significant scientific evidence illustrates the strong effect that salt intake in infancy and childhood has on predicting high blood pressure later in life.[27] The majority of Americans eventually require blood pressure medications; high sodium intake eventually takes its toll. One is typically considered sodium-sensitive if reducing salt intake shows a resultant decrease in blood pressure. Though it is easy to observe the effects of a high sodium intake and the resultant high blood pressure in sodium-sensitive individuals, apparently years and years of high sodium intake takes its toll as well on those who are not sodium-sensitive. It is difficult to discern which individuals are sensitive to the effects of a high-salt diet earlier in life because it takes many, many years to see the results.

A study that illustrates this appeared in the medical journal *Circulation*. The researchers studied a large group of high schoolers. In these adolescents they did not find a correlation of sodium intake with high blood pressure. But ten years later, the researchers could easily determine who had the high blood pressure by their early high levels of salt consumption. By reexamining the earlier records, they could see the strong correlation of sodium intake and higher blood pressure.[28]

Children who have been on a low-salt diet do not favor a high-salt diet later on. Those who develop the taste for a high-salt diet continue to prefer that throughout life.

Epidemiologic studies of populations with very low sodium intakes showed no hypertension in adults and the elderly in those populations with an average sodium intake of less than 1,350 mg per day. Keep in mind that there are pockets of Stone Age–like tribes around the world eating 100 percent natural foods that consume less than one gram of sodium daily. Natural foods generally contain approximately ½ mg of sodium per calorie. Primitive man lived in a salt-poor world. Only in the last few thousand years of human time on earth have humans had access to all the salt they desired.

Lowering sodium intake after high blood pressure develops does not have the same effect on reducing the occurrence of high blood pressure as would salt avoidance earlier in life. After reviewing hundreds of epidemiological, clinical, and experimental studies, leading scientists studying the effect between the intake of sodium and its long-term effect on blood pressure concluded, "There is strong, if not definitive evidence that reducing dietary salt intake to less than 2000 mg a day would eliminate hypertension as a major health problem."[29] The average American consumes approximately 4,000 mg of sodium per day. A diet of natural foods without added salt would typically contain an ideal level of sodium, between 600 and 1,000 milligrams of sodium per day.

THE OPTIMAL AMOUNT OF PROTEIN

Most of my patients tell me that the typical question their friends or family members have about eating a natural-food, plant-predominant diet style is, "How do I get enough protein with so little animal products in the diet?" Many people believe that a diet needs lots of animal products to be nutritionally sound. To add to the confusion are the diet books and magazine articles that promote a high protein intake at the expense of carbohydrates. Then there are those who argue that we should balance the precise ratio of fat, carbohydrate, and protein with a calculator or that we should determine the ideal macronutrient ratio based on our heritage, shoe size, eye color, blood type, or the spelling of our mother's maiden name backward. These trendy viewpoints are not scientifically valid and miss the critical issues in human nutrition. To understand human nutritional needs, it helps to first understand the difference between macronutrients and micronutrients.

Protein, fat, and carbohydrate are macronutrients, the only macronutrients that exist. Macronutrients are the nutrients that contain calories, thereby supplying us with energy. Micronutrients are those nutrients that don't contain calories, but have other essential roles to play. Examples of some micronutrients are vitamins, minerals, fiber, bioflavonoids, antioxidants, and other phytochemicals.

Unfortunately, modern societies eat diets deficient in micronutrients, but generally consume more macronutrients (calories) than needed. Indeed, that is one of the main problems: processed foods and animal products mostly contain macronutrients, but are deficient in micronutrients. We get too much protein, carbohydrate, and fat and insufficient micronutrients. This predicament promotes disease. Simply put, the goal of a healthy diet is to get the most micronutrients, both in amount and diversity, from the fewest calories (macronutrients).

Protein is ubiquitous; it is contained in all foods, not only animal products. Protein deficiency is not a concern for anyone in the developed world. It is almost impossible to consume too little protein, no matter what you eat, unless the diet is significantly deficient in calories and other nutrients as well.

Health problems arise when we consume more of something we are already getting enough of. Excesses hurt us, not just deficiencies, especially excesses of macronutrients. Studies have shown that as protein consumption goes up, so does the incidence of chronic diseases. Increases in carbohydrates and fat consumption have led to the same end result. If we need more calories and are chronically malnourished, like an anorexic, they are good, but they are all detrimental if we are already getting too much. If any of these nutrients exceed our basic requirements, the excess can be hurtful. Americans already get too much protein, especially too much animal protein. The simplest thing you can do to improve the diet of your family is to reduce protein and fat from animal-source foods and increase protein and fat from plant-source foods because of the high level of micronutrients contained in plant foods.

EATING MORE PLANT PROTEIN INCREASES
MICRONUTRIENT INTAKE

When you eat to maximize micronutrients, your body function will improve; chronic illnesses like high blood pressure, Type II diabetes, and high cholesterol will likely disappear; and your youthful vigor will last into old age. Heart disease and cancer, the major killers of modern societies, would fade away and be exceedingly rare occurrences if the population adopted a cancer-preventive diet style and lifestyle. And we would hardly ever see any overweight children.

Maintaining a population of normal-weight individuals can be efficiently accomplished only by eating more high-nutrient foods, foods with a higher nutrient-per-calorie ratio. The foods with the most nutrients per calorie are vegetables and beans. Vegetables are also very rich in protein and calcium. Most vegetables have more protein per calorie than meat and more calcium per calorie than milk. Nobody can consume too little protein by eating less animal products and substituting more vegetables, beans, nuts, and seeds.

The focus on the importance of protein in the diet is one of the major reasons we have been led down the wrong path to dietary suicide. We were taught to equate protein with good nutrition and have thought that animal products, not vegetables, whole grains, beans, nuts, and seeds, are our best source of protein. We bought a false bill of goods, and the dairy-and-meat-heavy diet brought forth a heart attack and cancer epidemic.

If we hear something over and over since we were young children, we just accept it as true. For example, it is a myth repeated over and over that plant proteins are "incomplete" and need to be "complemented" for adequate protein. In fact, all vegetables and grains contain all eight of the essential amino acids (as well as the 12 other nonessential ones).[30] While some vegetables have higher or lower proportions of certain amino acids than others, when eaten in amounts to satisfy one's caloric needs, a sufficient amount of all essential amino acids are provided. Because digestive secretions and sloughed-off mucosal cells are constantly recycled and re-absorbed, the amino acid composition in the bloodstream after meals is remarkably complete in spite of short-term irregularities in their dietary supply.

It is interesting to note that peas, green vegetables, and beans have more protein per calorie than meat. But what is not generally considered is that foods that are rich in plant protein are generally the foods that are richest in nutrients and phytochemicals. By eating more of these high-nutrient, low-calorie foods we get plenty of protein, and our bodies get flooded with protective micronutrients simultaneously. Animal protein does not contain antioxidants and phytochemicals, plant protein does. Plus, animal protein is married to saturated fat, the most dangerous type of fat.

PROTEIN CONTENT FROM SELECTED PLANT FOODS

Food	Grams of Protein
Almonds (3 oz)	10
Banana	1.2
Broccoli (2 cups)	10
Brown rice (1 cup)	5
Chickpeas (1 cup)	15
Corn (1 cup)	4.2
Lentils (1 cup)	18
Peas—frozen (1 cup)	9
Spinach—frozen (1 cup)	7
Tofu (4 ounces)	11
Whole wheat bread (2 slices)	5

Even a professional body builder who wants to build one-half pound of extra muscle per week only needs about an extra seven grams per day over a normal protein intake. No complicated formulas or protein supplements are needed to get sufficient protein for growth, even in the serious athlete. Exercise increases hunger, and as the athlete consumes more calories to meet the demands of exercise, they will naturally get the extra protein they need. Many world-class athletes thrive at world-class competitions on vegetarian and vegan diets.

When you reduce or eliminate animal protein intake and increase vegetable protein intake, you lower cholesterol radically. Vegetables, beans, and nuts and seeds are all rich in protein, and they also have no saturated fat or cholesterol. But the clincher is that they are higher in nutrients than any other foods. We must structure our diets around the foods that supply the most micronutrients.

The cholesterol-lowering effects of vegetables and beans (high-protein foods) are without question. When adult subjects are fed a vegetable-based diet, cholesterol levels drop radically, much more than with the most powerful cholesterol-lowering drugs.[31] These foods also contain an assortment of heart disease–fighting nutrients independent of their ability to lower cholesterol, and they fight cancer, too.

ARE ANIMAL PRODUCTS NEEDED FOR
EXTRA PROTEIN?

Animals eat their macronutrients; they don't fabricate them from the air. All protein, all fat, and all carbs are made from soil and water with energy from the sun via photosynthesis. Animals then get all the fat, protein, and carbohydrates for energy from plants. Amino acids are the building blocks of protein. All animals, directly or indirectly, receive protein (amino acids) from plants. The lion eats the antelope; the antelope got the protein it supplied to the lion from the grass. Green vegetables (the soil) supplied the nitrogenous compounds to make the protein for the antelope and ultimately the lion.

In North America, about 70 percent of dietary protein comes from animal foods. Worldwide, plants provide 84 percent of calories. In the 1950s human protein requirement studies were first conducted that demonstrated that adults require twenty to thirty-five grams of protein per day.[32] Today, the average American consumes 100 to 120 grams of protein per day, mostly in the form of animal products. People who eat a completely vegetarian diet (vegan) have been found to consume sixty to eighty grams of protein a day, well above the minimum requirement.[33] Vitamin B12, not protein, is the missing nutrient in a vegan diet.

In modern times, the plant foods we eat are well washed and contain little bacteria, bugs, or dirt, which would have supplied B12 in a more natural environment such as the jungle or forest. To assure optimal levels of B12 in our diet, we require some form of B12 supplementation when eating a diet with little or no animal products.

ARE MILK AND CHEESE NEEDED FOR CALCIUM?

When you eat a healthy diet rich in natural foods, fruits, vegetables, beans, nuts, and seeds, it is impossible not to obtain sufficient calcium. Of course, when our calories come mostly from oil, flour, and animal muscle parts (which have no calcium), instead of unrefined plant foods, it can appear that without dairy the diet would be too low in calcium. But the minute we remove the processed junk food, sugar, and oil from the diet, and instead encourage the consumption of natural foods such as nuts, seeds, fruits, and vegetables, we get the healthy fats we need, and we also get plenty of calcium.

To raise healthy children we need to reduce dairy fat and substitute more fats and more calcium from raw nuts and seeds, tofu, and vegetables. Today, both soy milk and orange juice are fortified with calcium and vitamin D. You do not have to be concerned about your children consuming too little calcium if you remove or reduce dairy.

Our body absorbs the calcium differently from different foods and absorbs calcium most efficiently from vegetables. Only about 32 percent of the calcium in milk is absorbed, while 54 percent of the calcium in bok choy is absorbed.

100 calories of	calcium	percentage and amount absorbed	
Skim milk	334 mg	32%	107 mg
Kale	449 mg	59%	265 mg
Bok choy	787 mg	54%	435 mg
Broccoli	189 mg	53%	100 mg

CALCIUM CONTENT OF COMMON FOODS

Almonds—raw	(½ cup)	180 mg
Broccoli	(1 cup)	180 mg
Milk (whole)	(1 cup)	291 mg
Navy beans	(1 cup)	140 mg
Orange	(2)	120 mg
Raisins	(½ cup)	60 mg
Sesame seeds	(¼ cup)	350 mg
Soybeans	(1 cup)	261 mg
Spinach	(1 cup)	244 mg
Tofu	(1 cup)	300 mg

When you eat less animal protein and less salt, you do not lose as much calcium in the urine and therefore need less calcium. Excess animal protein and sodium promote excessive calcium loss in the urine, increasing calcium requirements.[34] When you eat a diet predominating in natural foods the way nature designed them, you do not have to worry about getting extra calcium. In fact, more natural plant foods added to the diet (fruits and vegetables) have been shown to have a powerful effect on increasing bone density and bone health.[35] There are factors in these plants other than calcium that have beneficial effects on our bones. You and your child can achieve nutritional excellence utilizing a variety of natural foods while reducing dependence on dairy, and especially cheese and butter.

ENHANCING YOUR CHILD'S HEALTH IN THE KITCHEN

- Stock your home with a variety of produce—especially fresh fruits, raw vegetables, and raw nuts and seeds.

- Replace most foods of animal origin with foods of plant origin: bean burgers, vegetable/bean soups, and fruit-centered deserts. If using animal products, use only white-meat poultry and eggs a few times weekly and other animal products more infrequently.

- Make breakfast dishes, desserts, and sauces with raw nuts and seeds utilizing the recipes in chapter 5.

- Limit sweets and remove sugar, salt, and white flour from the home and all products with these ingredients.

- If eating dairy foods, select no-fat varieties such as fat-free milk. Reduce dairy consumption in general. Instead use nut milks, fortified soy milks, and orange juice, fortified with vitamin D. Cheese should not be kept in the home.

- As a time-saver, use a very large pot to make vegetable soups with beans so that the same soup can be used for days.

- Serve a cooked vegetable main dish every night.

two

Preventing and Treating Childhood Illnesses Nutritionally

Wouldn't it be terrific if we could eat anything we desired, party as much as we want, eat junk food all day, and never suffer the consequences? When we became sick, we could just go to this magical wizard, be given a pill, and immediately get well, and then we could start all over again. This make-believe world that most people think exists in reality is a fairy tale; Mother Nature is not that forgiving. Life is governed by the biological laws of cause and effect. We become what we eat, and our future health is dependent on how carefully we build our body with optimal nutrition and minimal exposure to dangerous chemicals and toxins.

Many people suffer with chronic illnesses: fibromyalgia, asthma, arthritis, colitis, multiple sclerosis, lupus, and many more dangerous and discomforting afflictions born from early life causes. Nevertheless, many keep looking futilely for a magical cure. Life can become difficult, not quite the fairy tale, after a childhood of inferior nutrition. A disease-free life can only be realized in an environment of healthful influences. Then life has the potential to reach all of its wonderful possibilities and like the fairy tale, we set the stage for our children to live happily ever after.

> Alli has been suffering from severe eczema since her first year of life. We had been to numerous specialists and tried many medical treatments to no avail. After two months on the diet you recommended, her condition has disappeared. The knowledge we have gained from your books has given us an incredible sense of freedom and control over our own health.
>
> —Majorie and Jim Webber

At the first pharmacology lecture I heard in medical school, the professor impressed on us that all drugs have toxicity and that it is our job as physicians to first do no harm. He established the foundation that medications are not the first resort; lifestyle and dietary modifications are. Later, I realized that very few physicians utilized lifestyle and dietary modifications to treat and prevent illness. It seemed as if I was the only one. I found that even the alternative practitioners were primarily involved with remedies and therapies, leaving the chief causes of illness uncorrected. We live in a pill- and remedy-oriented society. People are looking for a magic cure, rather than getting to the root cause of the problem.

Medical doctors, homeopaths, naturopaths, herbalists, Chinese medicine practitioners, Ayurvedic practitioners, and the like all give their favorite remedies as they fit their particular discipline. Receiving remedies does not necessarily make one healthier; in fact, they generally make one less healthy because they can add further toxic insult to the already weakened system.

Most health conditions are more effectively addressed by uncovering the causes that can be removed to allow the body's natural tendency to heal have free reign. Built into our genetic code is the ability to detoxify chemical compounds, remove wastes, heal defects, and repair injury. Our body is a remarkable self-repairing, self-healing marvel when the optimal environment for healing is put into place.

We can't smoke cigarettes with impunity, excessively consume alcohol without paying a price, or eat the typical American diet and not eventually develop atherosclerotic heart disease and cancer. Diseases have causes; avoiding the cause of disease is the best way to protect our valuable health. Symptoms are initiated by the body in order to remove the infectious or noxious agents and increase our body's natural defenses. Many substances, both natural and designed in the lab, have medicinal effects and can lessen the symptoms of disease. However, most such substances have such effects due to the presence of **noxious** compounds.

Whether the compound is derived from the willow bark tree or from the lab at Johnson & Johnson, substances that have pharmacologic effects are invariably nonnutritive substances that the body must attempt to eliminate before they can do damage to our pristine cells. Substances with therapeutic or medicinal effects, while they may be useful or even life-saving, do not make us healthier, and if consumed for a significant length of time can have negative effects on our long-term health.

This does not mean that herbal products and other remedies do not work; they can. However, they are harmful (toxic) in proportion to their power to act. You don't get something for nothing, and you can't gain excellent health by consuming medicinal substances or herbal remedies. Superior health is the result of nutritional excellence and healthy habits; it does not result from taking remedies. This does not mean that a natural substance with medicinal properties or even a drug should never be used, it means that we pay a price (a noxious stress to the body) from the use of such substances and we are better off if we can live in a manner to avoid such things.

Generally speaking, nutritive substances (vitamins, minerals, essential fatty acids, phytochemicals) have no specialized therapeutic effects. They merely make the body function normally. By supporting normal function, nutritional excellence increases our defenses against disease and prevents cellular damage that leads to disease.

SYMPTOMS—OUR DEFENSIVE RESPONSE AGAINST ILLNESS

Symptoms are the body's natural response to deal with the causes of disease, lessening their damage. Symptoms attempt to eliminate the cause of an illness, but are often mistaken for the illness itself. For example, when we get food poisoning, diarrhea is a beneficial response to wash away the offending microbes. Attempting to halt the diarrhea with medication is potentially harmful, as it may allow dangerous bacteria to proliferate and gain entry into the bloodstream. In acute illnesses, such as colds and flu, the symptoms such as fever, mucous production, and cough are the body's defenses to get rid of the virus. A fever promotes interferon production in the brain, which then further activates white blood cells to fight the virus. Coughing aids in expelling mucous, carrying away dead cells and preventing them from settling within the lungs.

Suppressing the fever and cough with medication can lead to a prolonged illness. In fact, cough suppressants and over-the-counter cold medicines expose children and adults to further drug side effects without significant effectiveness. We were taught in medical school that cough suppressants do not work well, which is good, because if the cough was really suppressed, the mucous would settle deep into the lung and cause pneumonia. The most common cough suppressants contain dextromethorphan and codeine. A head-to-head comparison between the placebo and these cough remedies showed that the placebo worked just as well. All children improved significantly by day three, and there was no difference among the three treatment groups in any symptom parameter.[1]

Self-medicating symptoms with over-the-counter medications may not be wise, but it can be more of a health risk to go to a doctor who, in response to patient demand, will provide an antibiotic. Antibiotics are useless against common viral illnesses. They are designed to treat the much more uncommon bacterial illnesses. Of course, antibiotics have their legitimate uses, but that would only encompass less than 10 percent of all antibiotics utilized in this country today.

When ill with a typical viral syndrome, it is best to rest, drink water, avoid cooked food, and only consume high-water-content fruits and vegetables if hungry. Avoid physicians, medications, and remedies. See a doctor only if the illness is unusual or unusually severe or prolonged. It would be a better idea to give antibiotics inappropriately to those who are well and not burden the sick people suffering with viruses with such potentially dangerous drugs.

NUTRITIONAL EXCELLENCE: AN ALTERNATIVE TO BOTH CONVENTIONAL AND COMPLEMENTARY MEDICINE

In the last thirteen years of my nutritionally oriented family practice it has been exceedingly rare that I have had to pick up a prescription pad. When put on my program of nutritional excellence, most of the children who had taken medication in the past no longer require it. I saw remarkable outcomes, watching young children recover from common illnesses such as:

- Asthma and allergies

- Attention Deficit Hyperactivity Disorder (ADHD)

- Constipation and digestive disturbances

- Ear infections (otitis media)

- Eczema and other common skin diseases

- Frequent illnesses and infections

I have seen children with juvenile rheumatoid arthritis who have made recoveries. One of my patients, a five-year-old girl, made a complete recovery from juvenile rheumatoid arthritis, without medication, in three months. Instead of taking the steroids and immunosuppressive drugs prescribed by her rheumatologist, she gleefully followed my dietary recommendations, and her swollen joints and high inflammatory markers in her blood slowly came back to normal.

ADHD AND DRUGS

The diagnosis and treatment of Attention Deficit Hyperactivity Disorder (ADHD) has skyrocketed in recent years, with a tremendous increase in the percentage of our elementary school children who are taking amphetamines and stimulants such as Ritalin, Adderall, Concerta, Cylert, and others. As many as 9 percent of school-age children show symptoms of ADHD such as inattention, hyperactivity, impulsivity, academic underachievement, or behavioral problems.[2]

These medications with their reported adverse effects and potential dangers were simply unnecessary for so many children whom I have seen as patients. I have witnessed consistently positive results when these children followed my comprehensive program of nutritional excellence. The scientific studies lending support to a comprehensive nutritional approach to treating ADHD are ignored by physicians, and drugs are generally the only method offered.

Most new cases of ADHD are of the inattentive subtype. Inattentive ADHD are the children who have a short attention span, are easily distracted, and can appear to be a brain fog; they do not have hyperactivity. Research on the use of psychostimulants in these patients has shown a high rate of nonresponders, and although medications showed a short-term decrease in symptoms, they did not improve grade point averages.[3]

Before a parent begins to consider the pros and cons of starting their inattentive child on stimulants such as Ritalin, they should give nutritional excellence a trial. Nobody knows for sure the long-term dangers of these stimulant drugs or if taking them for a long period of time during childhood increases one's later life risk of cancer. There certainly is some risk, especially because they can cause cancerous tumors in mice.[4]

The pertinent question is, why put your child at unnecessary risk, with the long-term use of drugs, when nutritional excellence is both effective, and not just safe, but also beneficial to their long-term health? Then you do more than improve your child's behavior; you improve the basic structure and function of his entire body, preventing the occurrence of other more serious, unrelated illnesses in the future.

The most widely studied dietary modification for the treatment of ADHD is the additive-free Feingold diet. This diet has been tested in numerous studies with variable results, and it is not very effective. Some studies where the researchers were blinded to which children were on a diet free of additives and food dyes show a small percentage of children demonstrating improvement in behavior, with approximately 5 to 25 percent of hyperactive children showing some benefit.[5] Clearly, this food-additive-free diet is a start and our children should not consume dyes and chemicals in their food, but eliminating them is not enough. Optimal brain function requires more than just removing food additives and food coloring in processed foods when the diet remains nutritionally poor and deficient in essential nutrients and essential fatty acids necessary for normal brain function. Simply eliminating refined sugar has also not been shown to be effective, either.

What has been shown to be highly effective in some recent studies is high-nutrient eating, removal of processed foods, and supplementation with omega-3 fatty acids.[6] The difference between my approach and others is that it changes a poor diet into an excellent one, supplying an adequate amount of thousands of important nutrients that work synergistically as well as removing those noxious substances such as chemical additives, trans fats, saturated fats, and empty-calorie food that place a nutritional stress on our brain cells. I believe this comprehensive approach is more effective; the scientific literature suggests this, and I have observed this in my practice with hundreds of ADHD children who have seen me as patients.

> George Grant, age eleven, is the nicest, most polite boy you would ever meet. Although his parents reported an improvement in his concentration and behavior since beginning Ritalin two years prior to his appointment with me, they were unsatisfied. George had frequent headaches and frequent stomachaches from the medication, and he had tried the other stimulant medications and found that the same problem occurred. I enjoyed meeting George and talking to him; he was surprisingly mature and interested in his school performance, and did not want his grades to suffer. I told them that it would take about three to six months to really evaluate whether nutritional intervention would work as effectively as the Ritalin, but one thing I could promise them: George would feel better, sleep better, have a better appetite, and his headaches and stomachaches would go away within a few weeks with high-nutrient eating. His parents were very happy when we were able to use less Ritalin over the next two months, and

then when George was on summer break he stopped taking his Ritalin completely. At school the following September, he was drug-free and performing better than he ever did on Ritalin. His parents sent me a copy of his report card, showing all A's and impressive comments from his teachers.

The causes of ADHD are complex and multifactorial. One contributing factor is excessive television watching early in life.[7] The findings that television watching early in life can affect brain function and shorten attention span supports the American Academy of Pediatrics' recommendation that youngsters under age two not watch television. ADHD can be prevented with early excellent nutrition, creative play, and minimizing exposure to television.

My successful outcomes, which I have observed in approximately 90 percent of the children I see for ADHD, does not involve any supplemental gymnastics, expensive blood tests, hair analysis, allergy workup, testing for toxic metals, or food diaries. I utilize a natural-food, high-nutrient dietary plan, just like the one I recommend to all my patients.

OMEGA-3 FATTY ACIDS AND DHA—NECESSARY FOR NORMAL BRAIN FUNCTION

Besides a multivitamin, the only other nutritional supplement I recommend for children with ADHD is additional DHA fat. Docosahexaenoic acid (DHA) is a long-chain omega-3 fatty acid. About half of the brain and eyes are made up of fat, much of which is DHA, which is an essential nutrient for optimal brain and eye function.[8] Children's diets today are notoriously low in the beneficial omega-3 fats found in foods such as walnuts, flax seeds, soybeans, leafy greens, and certain fish. I do not recommend fish as a preferred source of these beneficial fats for children because of contamination with pollutants and mercury.

The most commonly used supplement to add DHA to the diet is fish oils, but what is not widely known is that most of us can produce sufficient DHA from short-chain omega-3 fatty acids received from walnuts, flax seeds, and green vegetables. Many fish make their DHA from eating greens, too, from algae. Children prone to ADHD usually do not form as much DHA from the shorter omega-3 precursors found in nuts and seeds.

DHA is also a normal component of breast milk, and infants fed breast milk score higher on intellectual and visual measurements than those fed baby formulas lacking DHA. Children who were breast-fed, as a group, have higher IQ scores than those who were formula-fed.[9] Pregnant women should pay close attention to their DHA status to ensure proper DHA supply for prenatal development. Maternal supplementation with DHA during pregnancy, and lactation has been demonstrated to augment children's IQ.[10]

DHA is present in breast milk, but up until 2002, the United States was the only country in the world where infant formulas were not fortified with DHA, despite a 1995 recommendation by the World Health Organization to do so. In addition, the average DHA content of breast milk in the United States has been tested to be low compared to other countries that consume more fish. In fact, postpartum depression, lower IQ, dyslexia, and ADHD have been linked by many scientific studies to the low DHA intake common in the United States.[11]

DEFICIENCY IN DHA FATTY ACIDS HAS BEEN LINKED TO[12]

Impulsiveness	Sleep problems
Aggressiveness	Temper tantrums
Dyslexia	Alcoholism
Depression	Schizophrenia
Reduced Intelligence	Manic depression

An inadequate level of DHA fat has been demonstrated to be important in the etiology of many diseases, but especially in ADHD.[13] This important nutrient is typically found to be low in the blood of ADHD sufferers compared to other children without ADHD[14] and also has been found to improve the behavior and symptoms of ADHD. Therefore, supplementation is certainly indicated. I have done hundreds of blood tests checking the omega-3 and DHA status of children with ADHD. Almost every child brought to me with health complaints, eating the typical diet most kids in America eat, tests dangerously low in these essential fats.

It should not be any surprise to see signs of brain dysfunction in a growing number of America's children, especially when you consider that omega-3 fatty acid deficiency is only one common deficiency effecting health and brain dysfunction. Male animals generally require more DHA than females, and this may account for the increased incidence of ADHD in males. However, I am not suggesting that a DHA deficiency is the only factor creating a biological environment favorable for brain dysfunction; it is also a broad spectrum of nutritional inadequacies that potentiate abnormal brain chemistry.

DR. FUHRMAN'S ANTI-ADHD PLAN

Nutritional excellence combined with classroom and behavior modification for rewarding positive behavior is a promising approach for treating ADHD. Often family therapy is necessary as well to address behavioral, emotional, and self-esteem issues. Combined with a vegetable-based, high nutrient diet, great results are the norm, not the exception. The essential features of my dietary approach for ADHD are as follows:

- A high-nutrient, vegetable-nut-fruit–based diet

- One tablespoon of ground flax seeds daily, easily added to oatmeal, shakes, and desserts

- At least one ounce of raw walnuts daily, with the addition of other raw nuts

- DHA supplement of 100–600 mg daily

- No processed foods, no dairy fat, no trans fat

- Little or no oils; essential fats are supplied from raw nuts and seeds and DHA supplementation

- Some children also must avoid gluten (from wheat products) and/or casein (from dairy products), as they appear to be bothered by these frequently difficult-to-handle dietary proteins

Flax seeds and walnuts are rich sources of those beneficial but hard-to-find short-chain omega-3 fats, plus they are rich in lignans, minerals, and vitamins.

Until recently, the primary source of DHA dietary supplements was fish oil. However, new products are available that contain DHA from algae, the fish's original source. Unlike fish oils, the algae-derived DHA, grown in the laboratory, is free of chemical pollutants and toxins that may be present in some fish oil–based brands. I recommend favorable DHA products that are designed for purity and are suitable for children. Neuromins is a common (non-fish-derived) brand of DHA sold in most health food stores, and I also have designed and manufactured an all-plant-derived DHA supplement, available on my Web site and in my office.

To feed DHA-rich oil to a child is not difficult; just slice open the capsule with a serrated knife and mash it into a banana or mix it in orange juice or in morning oatmeal to disguise the taste. The dose may vary from 100 to 600 mg daily depending on the age and condition of the child. A child over the age of six with ADHD can be started on the higher dose for the first six months, and then the dose can be decreased to 400 mg daily for the next six months. I generally recommend supplementation with 100 mg of DHA to children six and under and 200 mg a day for seven and older. However, this dose should be doubled for those with ADHD until the symptoms resolve.

Many families who have adopted my diet of nutritional excellence, combined with judicious use of nutritional supplements, report that they begin to see improvement in as little as three months. Keep in mind, this nutritional approach to ADHD does not magically make the problem disappear overnight; it could take six months to observe a significant change in behavior. The chief factor that indicates a successful outcome is the entire family's willingness and desire to adopt a new healthy eating style for the benefit of all members. The child with the ADHD problem is never singled out as the only one required to eat healthy. In fact, I encourage the children to take responsibility in helping the parents to eat healthy, too. This prescription calls for nutritional excellence for the entire family. When families choose to work as a unit to improve the child's emotional environment and nutrition simultaneously, it is rare that psychostimulant medications are necessary.

INFECTIONS AND ANTIBIOTICS, AND MORE ANTIBIOTICS

When my child was eighteen months old and suffering from his fourth ear infection and fourth course of antibiotics, my search for a better solution led me to Dr. Fuhrman. After one visit, we changed my son's diet according to Dr. Fuhrman's instructions, and Evan never suffered another ear infection.

—Ondria Westfall

During the last ten years, the use of broad-spectrum antibiotics has gone up more than 50 percent in the United States.[15] As newer antibiotics are developed and marketed to doctors, they too often dispense the drugs without a legitimate clinical rationale for their use. Although there are instances when the use of antibiotics is appropriate, misuse can do long-term damage to your immune system.

Antibiotics are designed to kill bacteria; they do not kill viruses. Unfortunately, that is *not* how they are typically used. Approximately 90 percent of antibiotics are given for viral illnesses, against which they have no value. Antibiotics are routinely and repeatedly administered by physicians for illnesses such as colds and bronchitis, which are viral, not bacterial.[16] This use of antibiotics is inappropriate and dangerous. In one study, more than half of the patients who visited a physician in the United States with cold symptoms left with a prescription for an antibiotic.[17]

The misuse of antibiotics is a multibillion-dollar industry in the United States every year. Antibiotic therapy for the flu or acute bronchitis is also not supported by the scientific data. Patients do not benefit from antibiotics even in the presence of green or thick sputum, unless the person has chronic obstructive pulmonary disease (COPD), a disease primarily caused by smoking.[18] The color of the sputum was not found to be an indicator of bacterial involvement, as viral pathogens also produce thick, yellow- and green-tinted mucous. Besides their ineffectiveness, there are other compelling reasons to avoid antibiotics.

Antibiotics can cause diarrhea, digestive disturbances, yeast overgrowth, bone marrow suppression, seizures, kidney damage, colitis, and life-threatening allergic reactions. The unnecessary over-prescription of antibiotics during past decades has been blamed for the recent emergence of antibiotic-resistant strains of deadly bacteria. Besides these potential risks, in every single person who takes an antibiotic, the drug kills a broad assortment of helpful bacteria that live in the digestive tract and aid digestion. It kills the "bad" bacteria, such as those that can complicate an infection, but it also kills these helpful "good" bacteria lining your digestive tract that have properties that protect from future illness.

Nearly one-third of the dry weight of our stool is bacteria. Hundreds of different species of good bacteria play a very important role in your health by producing certain vitamins, such as B vitamins and vitamin K; they break down various fibers, and they produce other nutritive substances. For instance, these friendly flora make short-chain fatty acids (such as lipoic acid) and other nutrients that have antioxidant and immune-enhancing properties. In addition to these health-enhancing activities that enable your body to function more efficiently, these good bacteria secrete antibacterial substances that prevent the disease-causing bacteria from taking hold in your body.

Therefore, the presence of health-promoting bacteria crowds out and prevents the development of bacterial illnesses. When you eat a healthful, nutrient-rich, plant-based diet, you promote the growth of the right species of bacteria. For example, having a proliferation of the health-promoting species of bacteria is thought to offer protection against colon cancer. When you eat an unhealthful diet, it promotes the growth of microbes that can damage your health and body.

If you take antibiotics repeatedly when you are young, you further diminish the population of good bacteria that protects you against the harmful bacteria. In addition, the harmful bacteria become more resistant (harder to kill with antibiotics the next time).

Over 100 different helpful intestinal bacteria are lost with the use of antibiotics, which then give pathogenic (disease-causing) microbes and yeast the chance to proliferate and fill the ecologic vacuum created by the repeated administration of antibiotics.

Important Functions of Intestinal Microflora (Good Bacteria)

1. Supplements the digestive process to break down food.

2. Produces vitamins, short-chain fatty acids, and proteins utilized by the host.

3. Protects against overgrowth of pathogenic bacteria and yeast.

4. Strengthens immune function.

Harmful Effects of Pathogenic Bacteria and Yeast

1. Produce toxic substances, including carcinogens.

2. Harbor a reservoir of bacterial invaders to create future serious infections.

3. Produce digestive disturbances.

4. Promote immune system dysfunction and autoimmune inflammatory diseases.

Anyone who reads health news in newspapers and magazines knows that deadly bacteria are a growing threat to everyone. Hardly a week goes by without antibiotic-resistant bacteria turning up for every bacterial disease. Over 100,000 people die each year of hospital-acquired antibiotic-resistant infections. Antibiotics cause bacteria to mutate relatively quickly to develop resistance. The resistant bacteria can then transfer genetic material to nonresistant bacteria, causing them, too, to become resistant.

Repeated use of antibiotics can set the stage for recurrent infections and turn what might have started out as a minor illness into a more serious disease with a more virulent bacteria at a later date. Then, if an antibiotic is ever truly needed for a potential life-threatening infection, such as a bacterial pneumonia, it simply won't work anymore. People die daily from infections that were easily treated by antibiotics in the past; today the microbes are resistant.

The following hurtful cycle is all too prevalent today. We feed our children unhealthfully; they develop a cold, flu, bronchitis, or ear infection; we take them to a family physician or pediatrician who prescribes an antibiotic; and most of the harmful and the healthful bacteria are killed off. Without the helpful (good) bacteria they have become more susceptible to future infections and now harbor a colony of yeast and more virulent bacterial pathogens that survived the antibiotic. Another ear infection is now more likely, not less likely. The more antibiotics given, the more likely future bacterial infections will occur.

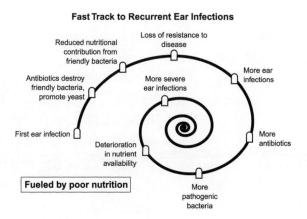

Fast Track to Recurrent Ear Infections

CHILDHOOD EAR INFECTIONS,
A MULTIBILLION-DOLLAR INDUSTRY

Ear infection, or otitis media, is the most common medical problem for children in the United States, and it is the most common reason for prescribing antibiotics for infants and children. Not only do nine out of ten children develop at least one ear infection each year, but almost one-third of these children develop chronic congestion with fluid in the middle ear that can lead to hearing loss and make the child a candidate for myringotomy, or tube placement by a specialist.

Babies who drink from a bottle while lying on their backs may get milk and juice into their eustachian tubes, which increases the occurrence of ear infections. Children who are breast-fed for at least a year have been shown to have much fewer infections than those weaned earlier.[19]

Studies also point to the fact that most ear infections early in life are viral, not bacterial.[20] The vast majority of ear infections resolve nicely on their own, whether bacterial or viral, without an antibiotic. It is common practice in this country to treat all ear infections with an antibiotic. Whether bacterial or not, our children get a routine prescription for an antibiotic at every minor illness. This cycle often is repeated many times, which may beget other medical problems in adulthood.

In some European countries, antibiotics are used for ear infections only when there is persistent drainage or persistent pain because these infections resolve on their own more than 85 percent of the time without treatment.[21] Studies show that the majority of ear infections are of viral etiology. For example, 75 percent of pediatric ear infections were caused by common respiratory viruses in a microbiologic survey.[22] Generally speaking, the use of antibiotics should be reserved for serious or life-threatening infections, not conditions that the body is well-equipped to resolve on its own. More and more physicians and authorities are recommending treating ear infections with antibiotics only when symptoms are not improving within three days and it is accompanied by drainage, fever, or persistent pain. Instead, eardrops for pain relief (available with a prescription) and other pain relievers can be used if the child is too uncomfortable to sleep.

A medical study reported on 168 children treated with antibiotics only if the illness followed an unusual course with high fever or profound weakness or if the child had a history of purulent meningitis or a concurrent serious bacterial infection. They followed up any children who did not recover in the typical time frame. As a result of their well-designed protocol, antibiotics were recommended by the physicians for only ten children, or less than 6 percent of all children presenting with acute ear infections. No serious complications, such as mastoiditis, meningitis, or permanent hearing loss, were observed.[23]

This is similar to the way I treat childhood ear infections, except that I also incorporate nutritional excellence, which I find dramatically reduces the likelihood of ever having an ear infection in the first place and then improves the likelihood of a quick recovery if illness does occur.

Another international study following over 3,000 children treated by general practitioners in nine countries showed that antibiotics did not improve the rate of recovery from ear infections. Nearly 98 percent of U.S. physicians in the survey prescribed antimicrobials routinely, the highest percentage of all countries surveyed.[24] The variable showing the strongest relationship with protection from ear infections was breast-feeding.[25]

Yet another double-blind study of fifty-three pediatric practices from the Netherlands placed half the children (aged 6 months to 2 years) with ear infections on placebo and the other half on ten days of amoxicillin. Parents kept a detailed symptom and outcome diary, all children were reexamined on day four and day eleven, and a researcher visited all children at home six weeks after treatment to collect information and perform tympanometry (measurement of eardrum mobility) and an ear exam. The median duration of fever was two days in the treatment group and three days in the placebo group. Similarly, symptoms resolved in a median of eight days in the treatment group and nine days in the placebo group.[26]

Ear infections early in life are generally a self-limited event during upper respiratory (viral) illnesses; they should not be routinely treated with antibiotics. The vicious cycle of poor nutrition and the overuse of antibiotics works to place a tremendous disease burden on the future health of our children. We bring our young (improperly fed) children to physicians with their first ear infection. At this point the majority of these infections are viral, not bacterial. Nevertheless, whether it's viral, bacterial, fungal, or some mixture, a healthy child has no problem recovering from an ear infection without antibiotics. In the United States almost all these children are routinely given antibiotics. Taking the antibiotic kills off the beneficial bacteria and promotes the colonization of more disease-causing strains, and now the next ear infection has a greater chance of being bacterial, not viral. Viral, bacterial, or a mixed infection, it matters not, because at the next visit your kid gets another antibiotic anyway, starting the cycle of infection after infection, antibiotic dependency, and impaired immune function.

The typical doctor does not take care to avoid the use of these dangerous drugs; he does not champion nutritional excellence to prevent future infections. The weak immune system from nutritional negligence leads to more frequent and more serious illness that is more difficult to recover from; then antibiotics complicate the issue and weaken the immune system further.

By the time Kyle was three, he had been on fourteen rounds of antibiotics for recurrent ear infections and it was recommended to us that we maintain Kyle on antibiotics indefinitely. Dr. Fuhrman put our entire family on his "therapeutic diet" with all the healthy fatty acids, and not only did Kyle stop having ear infections, but my other two children never had one again either.

—Joyce Brazinski

As a result of accumulating evidence documenting the dangers of antibiotics and their overuse, new guidelines for treating ear infections in children were just released from a joint effort of the American Academy of Family Physicians and the American Academy of Pediatrics. These guidelines represent a major shift in policy and thinking by physician leadership. The guidelines encourage doctors to initially manage the pain and not prescribe antibiotics for children who present with ear infections and to defer antibiotic use for the sicker children who are not improving two or three days later. I hope doctors will heed this message.

MORE AND MORE ANTIBIOTIC RISKS

The use of antibiotics in early childhood is also a contributor to the increasing incidence of allergies, asthma, and other problems. Medical studies have already linked a significant increased incidence of asthma, hay fever, and eczema to those receiving multiple antibiotic prescriptions early in childhood, especially in the first years of life.[27] A recent study involving more than 7,500 children showed that the number of ear infections earlier in life predicted the incidence of asthma down the road.[28] Children with a history of receiving multiple courses of antibiotics for ear infections were associated with higher parental education, likely reflecting greater access to medical care, where their children are routinely given antibiotics. The risk of wheezing and asthma rose as the number of antibiotic prescriptions given went up.

The association between pediatric antibiotic use and the later occurrence of Crohn's disease has been found in retrospective studies
that ask questions to patients with Crohn's about their prior use of
antibiotics. These studies utilizing questionnaires are not conclusive because they are susceptible to recall bias. *Recall bias* means the
answers may be colored by exaggeration or are given just to please
the investigator. However, recent prospective studies that followed
a large group of children over time and collected data on their use of
antibiotics and later on the incidence of diseases have confirmed the
findings of the earlier retrospective analysis; so lately more solid research is confirming this relationship.

Researchers have been hunting for clues because the incidence of
Crohn's disease has increased significantly over the last few decades.
There is increasingly persuasive evidence that the gut microflora are
intimately involved in the development of Crohn's and even other
autoimmune illnesses. In a review of 587 patients with Crohn's compared to 1,460 controls, researchers analyzed a computerized medical research database in England and reported a strong increased risk
for prior antibiotic users. Those with the disease had twice as many
antibiotic prescriptions in their past.[29]

Not only is the toxicity of the antibiotics themselves a problem,
but destruction of the body's beneficial flora may play a role in increasing the risk of cancer. A case-control study tracked 2,266 women
with invasive breast cancer and 7,953 randomly selected women to
function as the control group. Antibiotic use was tracked from
computerized pharmacy records. This study, published in the
Journal of the American Medical Association, found that women who
had more than twenty-five prescriptions for antibiotics over a
seventeen-year period had more than twice the risk of breast cancer
as women who had not taken any antibiotics. The risk was smaller
for women who took antibiotics for fewer days. However, even
women who had between one and twenty-five prescriptions over
an average period of seventeen years were about 1.5 times more

likely to be diagnosed with breast cancer than women who didn't take any antibiotics. This increased risk was observed for all classes of antibiotics.[30]

Young children, because of their developing immune systems and rapidly dividing cells, are more sensitive to the toxic side effects of drugs and antibiotics. There are no innocuous treatments. Besides the usual side effects adults get, children suffer from adverse effects uniquely common to children.[31]

> When Stephanie Rogers, a typical seven-year-old girl, became my patient, her parents handed me a printout from the local pharmacy documenting the filling of sixty-seven rounds of antibiotics at the cost of $1,643.80 by the ripe age of seven. Once the pediatric group started prescribing antibiotics for minor complaints of fever and cough, it escalated to ear infections, sinus infections, and finally visits to the ear specialist by the age of four. She received fifteen separate prescriptions of antibiotics when she was five years old. The first year she was my patient, the entire family changed their diet style. Stephanie went along for the ride and did fine. I did use an antibiotic once for her that next winter, when she had a persistent high fever and a red painful eardrum; however, that was the last time an antibiotic prescription was necessary. Luckily, Stephanie has been free of antibiotics ever since.

The U.S. Centers for Disease Control and Prevention has been asking physicians for years to be more prudent when prescribing antibiotics in order to help lower the incidence of dangerous antibiotic-resistant bacteria. Our antibiotic arsenal is becoming ineffective when a life-threatening illness is on the line because of unnecessary and excessive prescribing by physicians.

But what is not generally recognized, as to why children are chronically susceptible to so many infections, is their marginal nutritional status, which weakens their defenses. Breast-feeding for close to two years along with a diet of natural foods is the most effective way to keep your children away from medication in early life. It is not just luck that my own four children have never had, and those I care for in my medical practice rarely develop, ear infections and persistent bacterial illnesses.

Fortunately, the healthy human body has a tremendous capacity to fight and recover from diseases without antibiotics. The recovery may be somewhat slower when the body is allowed to heal itself, but the healing usually will be more complete. Not only will a healthier, better-nourished child be more likely to resist disease, but the well-nourished child is more resistant to complications and serious problems from the microbe.

STREP THROAT MUST HAVE
AN ANTIBIOTIC, RIGHT?

Pharyngitis, or sore throat, accounts for a significant proportion of antibiotic use today. More than 75 percent of those with sore throats are given antibiotic prescriptions by their physicians in spite of the fact that only about 10 percent are caused by bacteria in adults and about 30 percent in children. About half of all children with positive cultures showing strep actually have an acute infection; the other half represent a carrier state. Some children who always test positive for strep chronically "carry" a small amount of the bacteria, but it does not make them sick and they do not pass it on to others. If carefully tested to control for all children who are chronic carriers and always test positive, doctors would find that only 15 percent of sore throat patients have a strep throat worthy of treatment.

Although sore throats are self-limited and it is extremely rare to develop any long-term ill effects, physicians report that they prescribe antibiotics knowing they are not necessary. Doctors report that they do so in order to meet patients' expectations, so as not to disappoint parents looking to give their child something. This is hardly a reason to give a potentially dangerous prescription to an unsuspecting toddler who was never informed that these drugs might damage his health later on.

Never give your child an antibiotic for a sore throat unless it has been tested for strep and came back positive. Doctors cannot tell by examining the child if a sore throat is caused by strep or not; it must be tested.

It is an almost universally accepted practice to give antibiotics to all who are tested and found to harbor Group A beta-hemolytic strep. Diagnosing a strep throat is the major objective of the doctor visit when one has a sore throat, as it is thought that it is necessary to treat this type of sore throat to prevent dangerous aftereffects from strep, such as rheumatic fever or complications involving the kidney.

The question has to be asked, which is more risky to our children, treating strep throat with antibiotics to reduce the probability of rheumatic fever occurring later, or not treating strep throat because the possible long-term damage from treating so many with antibiotics exceeds the problems that might have developed if not treated? This is a difficult question to answer, and I do not claim to have the definitive answer, but nevertheless, we must consider the question, especially in light of the documented dangers of our present practice of raising our children on so much antibiotics.

It is important to consider more of the data before we make up our minds. First of all, no physician believes it is necessary to treat viral sore throats or other strains of bacteria causing sore throats because they resolve on their own. Second, we know that Group A strep resolves in a short period of time, too, if left alone and not treated. If physicians do not treat strep throats to make people get better, they will get better anyway. The rationale to treat strep throats (as we were taught) is to prevent the long-term damage that can very rarely occur about a month after the strep throat is gone. Physicians and health authorities are concerned about rheumatic heart disease and glomerulonephritis (kidney damage) if the strep infection is left to resolve naturally. We were taught that antibiotics will prevent outbreaks of rheumatic heart disease and that doctors save lives by testing and treating all the strep throats we find. Do we?

First, consider that there is no solid evidence that antimicrobial therapy decreases the incidence of post-streptococcal glomerulonephritis, which is very rare even in the absence of antibiotic treatment. The only legitimate rationale to treat strep is the prevention of rheumatic heart disease that can result from acute rheumatic fever.

However, because of repeatedly low and unchanging reported rates of acute rheumatic fever in the last ten years, the Centers for Disease Control dropped this disease from active national surveillance in 1994. In 1993, there were 112 cases of acute rheumatic fever nationwide and none in most East Coast states. This is in spite of the fact that the majority of children with sore throats never see a physician and the majority of strep throats are never diagnosed and treated.

The strains of strep prevalent in the past that were linked to rheumatic fever are simply very uncommon today. The strain of Group A beta-hemolytic strep associated with rheumatic fever has declined to the point that we have no idea how many, if any, cases of rheumatic fever are being prevented with antibiotics. There has been a decrease in the rheumatogenic potential of streptococcal strains, so luckily strep doesn't cause rheumatic

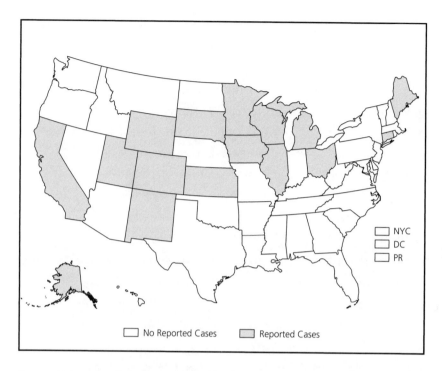

☐	NYC
☐	DC
☐	PR

☐ No Reported Cases   ■ Reported Cases

Source: U.S. Dept. of Health and Human Services. Centers for Disease Control and Prevention. "Summary of Notifiable Diseases, United States, 1993." Morbidity and Mortality Weekly Report (MMWR) *1994; 42(53): 48.*

heart disease like it used to. We don't know if any rheumatic heart disease is actually being prevented by all the thousands of antibiotic prescriptions handed out to young children every hour.

Treating so many sore throats with antibiotics may be causing more damage than benefit. Keep in mind, 70 percent of all sore throats, most of which are not strep, are treated with antibiotics. Until evidence is available documenting the prevention of glomerulonephritis or that antibiotic use is responsible for preventing a significant number of rheumatic fever cases in today's extremely low climate of rheumatic occurrence, I even question the current standard of practice of treating documented strep throats with antibiotics. There are not sufficient studies to accurately measure the long-term morbidity and suffering caused by all the antibiotics given to our young children, nor are there sufficient studies documenting the occurrence of rheumatic heart disease in an untreated population. At this point, nobody knows for sure. We must weigh the decision to use antibiotics carefully, especially when we are alerted to the possibility of immune system disorders, lifelong allergies, and cancer being caused by antibiotic use in the early years of life.

I hope in the near future the Centers for Disease Control resumes the reporting of all cases of acute rheumatic fever and advises physicians accordingly if more cases are noted in areas of the country. They could issue physicians periodic advisements on whether the strain of Group A beta-hemolytic streptococcus that is linked to rheumatic fever has been found in the state in which they live, so that an informed decision can be made about treating strep throats or not. This informed decision is ultimately the responsibility of an informed parent in consultation with their doctor. But one thing we know for sure: doctors must alter their present liberal prescribing practices—they are dangerous.

ASTHMA AND ALLERGIES

Asthma is an inflammatory disorder of the lungs that has skyrocketed in incidence and mortality worldwide in recent years, doubling within the last thirty years in children. Suffering and deaths continue to rise in spite of declines in air pollution. An amazing 16 percent of children develop asthma, according to a 2001 survey from the Centers for Disease Control and Prevention.

Allergies and asthma are often a reaction to inhaling irritating substances such as pollen, house dust, and cat hair, or the hyperreactivity of the airways may be triggered by infections, chemical irritants, exercise, and even emotions. In virtually every case, there is an underlying abnormality—an excessive irritability of the airways that leads to inflammation and narrowing of the airways.

It is always prudent to avoid and remove things that are known to trigger a reaction in a sensitive child, but what is more important, but rarely even considered, is why an individual is so hypersensitive or allergic to begin with. Learning why a person has allergies or asthma makes it possible to take steps to improve and reverse this common chronic condition.

The occurrence of asthma and allergies is also related to lifestyle factors and dietary patterns. Genetics play a role, but not the major role. Children's growing bodies and dividing cells make them more susceptible to damage, but there is an up side, too. Their growing bodies are also more malleable and can make dramatic recoveries from serious diseases such as asthma easier than an adult's can, when a program of superior nutrition is adopted.

Certainly, living in an urban area around pollution is an important contributor. Nondietary risk factors include exposure to day care before four months of age, and exposure to wood smoke, oil smoke, or exhaust anytime from birth to age five all increased asthma risk by 50 percent.[32] But nutritional influences are also powerfully linked and appear again and again in multiple scientific studies. One important risk for the development of allergies and asthma is lack of breast-feeding and high dietary ratio of omega-6 fatty acids to omega-3 fatty acids.[33] Animal products (except for fish) are deficient in omega-3 fatty acids, while flax seeds and walnuts are rich plant sources of omega-3 fats. This same inadequate dietary fatty acid pattern in the mother's diet during pregnancy has also been shown in scientific trials to beget a higher number of allergic and asthmatic children.[34]

Eating protein-rich and fat-rich foods of animal origin—meat, cheese, fried food, and saturated fat—is associated with a higher prevalence of both allergies and asthma.[35] Eating in fast food restaurants and eating a lower intake of vegetables and other fiber-rich foods has been implicated by numerous studies. The same studies also show that the children in the lowest third of vitamin E intake were found to have three times the incidence of asthma compared to those children in the highest third of vitamin E intake.[36] Vitamin E is a fat-soluble vitamin found in greens, raw nuts, and seeds; it is not found in animal products. The consumption of white bread, butter, and margarine has also been noted to be strongly associated with asthmatic symptoms.[37]

The same pattern emerges. What is needed to battle the development of asthma and allergies is the same adequate intake of omega-3 fat as well as a diet rich in fruits and vegetables. Eating high antioxidant- and phytochemical-containing foods is related to lower occurrence of childhood allergies and asthma.[38] Nutritional excellence can normalize an excessive inflammatory response. The inflammatory cascade releases chemicals that attract white blood cells and fluid into the area, which results in the tightness and swelling that create the symptoms of asthma. When nutrient intake is low, the lung tissues become overly sensitive to irritating stimuli.

Jonathan was an eight-year-old third-grader who developed asthma when he started first grade two years earlier. He was seen by his pediatrician and given a nebulizer, and later inhaled steroids, to deal with recurrent episodes of wheezing and the inability to exercise and play without fatigue and breathing difficulties. Jonathan was an excellent student and was keenly interested in learning how what he ate effected his health and his breathing problem. At the initial visit to my office,

Jonathan was instructed on using a spacer with an inhaler and he was taken off his three times a day nebulizer treatments. I told him his recovery hinged on the amount of green vegetables he was capable of eating. He was more than cooperative. This eight-year-old said to me, "I will eat dirt if you can fix my breathing." So I said, "How about if I give you great-tasting real food to fix your asthma? You can be a lot better within a year." Jonathan is now in fourth grade. It took about eight months until he no longer required any medication. He is now the picture of health and uses no inhalers or other asthma medications.

My experience working with asthmatic children has demonstrated that nutritional excellence enables the asthma to resolve in a predictable time frame and can routinely resolve even in cases when the allergies and asthma could be considered severe.

Jeff and Brian were twin brothers who both had severe allergic reactions. Soy milk, cow's milk, peanuts, corn, strawberries, cats, and dogs, in fact, almost anything set them off with severe skin rashes and breathing difficulties. They came to the office many times with severe illnesses, raw eczematous skin, and breathing difficulties. It seemed they required daily treatment with inhaled asthma nebulizers just to survive. They were my patients since they were three years old. With my guidance, their parents worked very hard to raise them in a clean environment with little exposure to dust mites and, of course, no cats. They took fatty acid nutritional supplements and ate a very healthy diet. By the time they were five, they had only occasional wheezing when they suffered with a viral illness, and by the time they were seven, their allergic condition had totally resolved. I can't prove their upbringing with superior nutrition resolved their very strong allergic tendencies, but it seems pretty likely that their eventual recovery and excellent health was the result of their wonderful efforts at superior nutrition.

These cases do not constitute a double-blind study, but when you consider the overwhelming evidence in the scientific literature and then apply that knowledge to real kids with medical difficulties, you see lots and lots of great kids who have made impressive recoveries from their allergies and asthma after a year or two of nutritional intervention.

Dietary Guidelines for Children with Allergies and Asthma

- A high-nutrient, vegetable-nut-fruit-based diet

- One tablespoon of ground flax seeds daily

- At least one ounce of raw walnuts daily, with the addition of other raw nuts

- DHA supplement, 100–400 mg daily

- Multivitamin without vitamin A or isolated beta-carotene

- No processed foods, dairy fat, or trans fat

- Little or no oils; essential fats are supplied from raw nuts and seeds and DHA supplementation

- Avoidance of known allergens

MILK, CHEESE, AND WHEAT—FREQUENT PARTNERS IN CRIME

A large number of children have marginal intolerances to wheat and other gluten-rich flours. If your child is frequently ill, chronically congested, or suffers from digestive complaints, it would be wise to try to reduce or eliminate most gluten-containing flours and see if you note a significant improvement.

However, the leading cause of digestive intolerance leading to stomach complaints is dairy products. Many kids have subtle allergies to cow's milk that perpetuate their nasal congestion, leading to ear infections. Cow's milk protein is the leading cause of food allergies in children.[39] Also, many children are lactose-intolerant. Seventy percent of blacks, and 90 percent of Asians, and 50 percent of Hispanics do not digest milk sugars well.

Milk, which is designed by nature for the rapidly growing cow, has about half its calories supplied from fat. The fatty component is concentrated more to make cheese and butter. Milk and cheese are the foods Americans encourage their children to eat, believing them to be healthy foods. Fifty years of heavy advertising by an economically powerful industry has shaped the public's perception, illustrating the power of one-sided advertising, but the reality and true health effects on our children is a different story.

Besides the link between high-saturated-fat foods (dairy fat) and cancer, there is a body of scientific literature linking the consumption of cow's milk to many other diseases. If we expect our children to resist many common illnesses, they simply must consume less milk, cheese, and butter. Dairy foods should be consumed in a limited quantity or not at all.

Childhood diabetes is an important consideration. Data from a multicountry analysis of cow's milk consumption showed a strong correlation between milk consumption in children and the incidence of childhood-onset (Type 1) diabetes.[40] As the consumption of cow's milk increased in a country, so did the incidence of childhood-onset diabetes. Many researchers in this field believe the causality of this disease is related to the consumption of cow's milk proteins early in life, before the digestive tract has fully matured.

The theory implicating cow's milk as a contributory factor in the causation of Type 1 diabetes is that susceptible children produce antibodies to cow's milk proteins and these antibodies cross-react and destroy the beta cells in the pancreas that produce insulin. Multiple studies have demonstrated that children with insulin-dependent diabetes have higher levels of cow's milk protein antibodies.[41] It is theorized that a viral illness may trigger this increased immune system response in milk-drinking kids.

An important point in this cow's milk and diabetes link is that children given cow's milk–based formula in the first three months of life were found to be 52 percent more likely to develop the disease than those not consuming cow's milk proteins. Even though exposure to cow's milk proteins during infancy greatly increases the risk of diabetes, drinking large amounts of cow's milk after infancy has also been shown to increase risk. Lack of breast-feeding and exposure to other food proteins too early, such as eggs or wheat, could also be contributory.[42] Coming on the heels of a meta-analysis of twenty other studies that reached the same conclusion, researchers such as Hans-Michael Dosch, M.D., professor of pediatrics and immunology at the Hospital for Sick Children in Toronto, stated, "the suspected link is now very solid."[43]

Diseases with Strong Links to Cow's Milk

1. Allergies[44]

2. Anal fissures[45]

3. Childhood-onset (Type 1) diabetes

4. Chronic constipation[46]

5. Crohn's disease[47]

6. Ear infections[48]

7. Heart attacks[49]

8. Multiple sclerosis[50]

9. Prostate cancer[51]

Crohn's disease is a chronic debilitating inflammatory disease of the bowel with an increasing incidence in modern societies. Accumulating evidence has implicated a bacterium that is transmitted via pasteurized cow's milk in the etiology of this tragic disease. It was discovered that a bacterium called *Mycobacterium avium paratuberculosis* (MAP) found in dairy products survives the heat of pasteurization and causes inflammatory bowel disease in a variety of animals, including monkeys and chimpanzees. In the last few years, this same bacterium has been detected in a large percentage of humans who have Crohn's disease.[52] To quote the most recent of these referenced medical journal articles, "The rate of detection of Mycobacterium avium subspecies paratuberculosis in individuals with Crohn's disease is highly significant and implicates this chronic enteric pathogen in disease causation."

An unexpected finding from all this research on Crohn's disease was the revelation that patients suffering from **irritable bowel syndrome** may also be affected with MAP from dairy product consumption.[53] The problems caused by the MAP bug, transmitted from dairy products, may be a severe public health issue, as millions of people suffer with these unfortunate diseases.

Cow's milk contains the calcium people need, but other foods are rich in calcium, too, including vegetables, beans, nuts, and seeds. Today we do not need to rely on cows for our calcium. We can eat greens directly for calcium, the place where cows get it to begin with, and orange juice and soy milks are fortified with calcium and vitamin D, too. It is easy to meet our nutrient needs for these substances without the risks of cow's milk.

It is better if young children are weaned from the breast onto a diet of mostly real food. Many of today's children utilize cow's milk as their leading source of calories. That is why milk is the most common cause of iron-deficiency anemia in infants and young children. Milk is deficient in iron, and it can also bind with the iron that is found in other foods, preventing iron absorption. The inflammatory reaction against milk that often occurs in infants and toddlers can also cause microscopic bleeding in their digestive tracts, leading to blood loss and anemia. Human breast milk is perfectly designed for little humans. Cow's milk is perfectly designed for the baby cow.

The antibodies derived from mother's milk are necessary for maximizing immune system function, maximizing intelligence, and protecting against immune system disorders, allergies, and even cancer. The child's immune system is still underdeveloped until the age of two, the same age when the digestive tract seals the leaks (spaces between cells) designed to allow the mother's antibodies access to the bloodstream. So picking the age of two as the length of recommended breast-feeding is not just a haphazard guess, it matches the age at which the child is no longer absorbing the mother's immunoglobulins to supplement his own immune system. Nature designed it that way.

Breast-feeding for two years might be considered a prolonged time by today's standards, but this practice offers significant protection against childhood diseases, including allergies and asthma. One recent study showed that breast-feeding for less than 9 months was found to be a risk factor for asthma and after that period of time, the longer the child was breast-fed, the lower the risk of asthma.[54] Avoiding cow's milk proteins, even those found in infant formulas, has also been shown to reduce asthma occurrence.[55]

A child is mostly eating solid food after one year of age, but it is a good idea to continue with some breast-feeding even if just twice a day until the second birthday. After weaning from the breast, the same qualities that make a healthy adult diet, a diet rich in fruits, vegetable, beans, nuts, and seeds, make the best diet for children.

The bottom line is to have your children develop a taste for other wholesome drinks besides cow's milk. Try soy milk or almond milk, or a mix of soy and almond. Many options are available fortified with vitamin D, vitamin B12, and calcium. If using dairy products or milk, stick to the fat-free variety. The fat in our children's diet should mostly come from avocadoes, nuts, and seeds, not cows.

three

Understanding the Causes of Cancer and Other Illnesses

It was not until after World War II that the emphasis on human nutrition research shifted from vitamins and mineral deficiencies to the association between diet and chronic disease and cancer. Interest in the role of diet, nutrition, and cancer increased rapidly during the 1960s, when the World Health Organization examined diet and lifestyle factors and concluded that the majority of human cancers are preventable.[1]

Data collected in the last forty years have generally come to the same conclusion: a high-calorie, high-fat, low-fiber, low-nutrient diet increases cancer risk at all ages. An increasing number of scientific organizations in the United States—including the National Cancer Society, the American Cancer Society, and the Department of Health and Human Services—support this conclusion and have issued dietary guidelines for the general public aimed at reducing the risk of cancer as well as other chronic diseases.

Although the evidence linking diet to cancer is strong, for some reason the fundamental lessons learned over the last forty years through scientific research have not filtered down to the public or created significant dietary modifications in our population. Cancer incidence has changed little. The economic power of big business to advertise, lobby government, and exert political clout, combined with social forces that favor the status quo, have blunted the message. Food advertisements, food industry press releases, and the favored status that money buys in the media and government have worked. Modern societies have headed down the path to obesity, diabetes, heart disease, and cancer.

A plethora of scientific information remains hidden from the general public. Instead, we are offered a more socially acceptable viewpoint via the news media, magazines, and books that genetics governs the occurrence of disease and that seeing physicians for detection and treatment is the preferred method of dealing with disease.

Cancer poses a great risk to those in the modern world, and that risk has not decreased. If you are a woman, you have a 38 percent lifetime risk of developing cancer. If you are a man, your chances are even worse—you have a 45 percent chance.[2] What is the answer to these alarming statistics? Is it to invest billions of dollars in the development and testing of more drugs to treat cancer patients, or is it to take some of those resources and educate the population to avoid the causes of cancer? I believe that instead of focusing our efforts on treating the symptoms of cancer in those who already have it, we must understand the causes of cancer and change ourselves and our environment to protect our future and the future of our loved ones.

The concept that we are in control of our own health destiny as a result of what we eat is discussed in scientific research papers but has not been appreciated by the medical profession or made widely known to the general public. As a result of this lack of awareness, we are a nation suffering from premature degenerative and life-shortening diseases. We are also burdened by escalating health care costs. We futilely attempt to deal with the tragic consequences of poor nutrition too late.

Excluding the high rate of lung cancer in smokers, the two most prevalent cancers in modern societies are breast and colon cancer in women, and prostate and colon cancer in men. Both the incidence of and the death rate from these common cancers have shown no significant decrease between 1930 and today. In other words, modern cancer detection and treatment methods have not changed the percentage of people dying from these common cancers.[3]

Clearly, it is time to direct our attention to the cause of disease. Cancer is more effectively prevented than treated. If we take a careful look at the scientific evidence, there is no doubt that the most powerful weapon we have to defeat the current epidemic of cancer deaths is nutritional excellence, started early in life.

CONFLICTING SCIENTIFIC STUDIES

Dietary practices have been implicated in the causation and incidence of the most common cancers. The countries with the highest incidence of cancers of the digestive tract, breast, and prostate are in

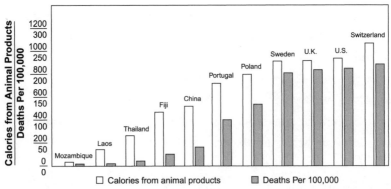

Breast and Prostate Cancer Deaths correlated with Animal Product Consumption

(55–85 age range)

Sources: Data compiled from World Health Organization Statistical Information System (http://www3.who.int/whosis/mort/table1.cfm?path=whosis,mort,mort_table1&language=english) and Food and Agriculture Organization of the United Nations (http://faostat.fao.org/faostat/default.jsp?language=EN&version=ext&hasbulk=0).

North America, Western Europe, and Australia, while in contrast the occurrence is lowest in Southeast Asia.[4] For example, when compared to the United States, Laos, Cambodia, and Thailand have only one-twentieth the amount of these three cancers in the fifty-to-seventy-five age bracket. Breast and prostate cancer are the most prevalent cancers in America.

The huge geographic variability in the incidence of these cancers suggests dietary factors as the main cause. It is believed that the diets that are lower in animal products, lower in saturated fat, and higher in unrefined plant foods account for these dramatic differences. When people from a low-risk country migrate to the United States, their cancer rate increases considerably and the cancer rate in their offspring jumps up to match that of other Americans. This demonstrates that the lower incidence of these cancers is not due to a lower genetic susceptibility in Asians, but rather to the exposure to Western dietary practices.[5]

Fat, particularly animal fat, has been implicated as a cause of cancer by hundreds of studies, while the high consumption of fruits and vegetables has been shown to protect against all forms of cancer.[6] These epidemiologic studies look at the differences in lifestyle and dietary patterns between populations with high cancer rates and those with low cancer rates. Data from studies on laboratory animals also implicate omega-6 oils and saturated fat intake as powerful cancer promoters.[7]

Epidemiologic Studies Tell Us

- Saturated fat is a powerful cancer promoter.

- Refined sugar and white flour promote cancer.

- Root vegetables and whole grains offer minimal cancer protection.

- Unrefined plant foods (UPF), fruits, vegetables, nuts, seeds, and beans are powerful cancer protectors.

The largest and most impressive epidemiologic study was the China Project. The *New York Times* called this investigation the *"Grand Prix of all epidemiologic studies"* and *"the most comprehensive large study ever undertaken of the relationship between diet and the risk of developing disease."*[8]

The reason this large undertaking, involving hundreds of researchers from Cornell and Oxford universities, produced such respected data is because China was the perfect test tube, "a living laboratory," to detect the effects food has on the incidence of different cancers. The people in one small area of China eat a certain diet, while just 100 miles away they may eat a vastly different one. The investigators were able to study populations with a broad range of dietary differences. In addition, the Chinese individuals who were tested had lived their entire lives in the same town, and therefore the dietary effects were present for the subjects' entire lives. In America, there is comparatively little difference in diet from one city to the next.

This project reported disease rates from towns that ate almost a complete plant-based diet and from other areas that ate a significant amount of animal products. The researchers found that as the amount of animal products increased in the diet, even in relatively small increments, so did the emergence of the types of cancers that are common in the West. The researchers noted that most cancers increased in direct proportion to the quantity of animal products eaten and decreased relative to the amount of fruits, vegetables, and beans consumed.

The more animal products in the diet, the greater the cancer occurrence.

The more fruits and vegetables in the diet, the less cancer they found.

Areas of China with exceptionally low intakes of animal products were virtually free of the cancers and heart disease that develop
in most people living in Western countries. Even lean meats, chicken,
eggs, and wild and naturally raised livestock (without hormones
and antibiotics) were shown to increase the heart attack and cancer
rates in proportion to the amount consumed by the population under study. Green vegetable consumption showed a strong protective
effect.[9]

THE FLY IN THE OINTMENT

Hundreds of epidemiologic studies have generated a huge body of
evidence that points to the fact that a dietary pattern high in animal
products and low in fruits and vegetables is evident in populations
with high cancer rates. This dietary pattern is prevalent worldwide
in the so-called "developed" countries. What has thrown a monkey
wrench in this clear-cut pattern are the case-control and cohort
studies done in the last twenty years. The cohort studies did not
confirm the results of the epidemiologic studies, creating confusion
and doubt. Individuals have used the results of the cohort studies as
reason to suggest that diet does not matter.

Epidemiologic studies look at populations with varying
characteristics for comparison.

Case control studies compare two groups: one with the
disease in question, and one group without. Past food intake
is determined by the use of questionnaires.

Cohort studies follow two groups over time, looking for
differences that appear years later.

Case control studies have shown an association with animal fat consumption and cancer, but this is not considered convincing evidence, as patients with cancer have a tendency to exaggerate their prior fat intake on diet recall questionnaires.

The cohort studies are more respected because they follow separate groups over a long time period, collecting accurate data. The cohort studies have not shown a clear-cut relationship between dietary fat (even saturated fat) and cancers of the breast, prostate, and colon or have only shown a moderate relationship.[10] The Nurses Health Study showed that American women who reduced their fat intake did not see a decreased incidence of breast cancer.[11]

Why do the epidemiologic studies and the cohort studies show different results? Do these conflicting results mean that saturated fat is not a significant risk factor for cancer? Is a high-fiber diet that includes large amounts of natural, unrefined plant foods such as fresh fruit, raw nuts and seeds, vegetables, and beans not protective? Is the huge amount of data collected in the China Project and other convincing epidemiologic studies wrong?

The cohort studies performed on adults lend argument to those denying the diet cancer link. They are touted by proponents of high-fat diets that are rich in animal products as evidence that animal products do not cause cancer. But the question remains, why do these studies not reveal the same data as the preponderance of the best epidemiological studies?

Because all the epidemiological studies can't be wrong, there are two possibilities. The first possibility is that these cohort studies followed adults who are past the age when diet plays a significant role. The middle-aged adults who attempted to eat more carefully to prevent cancer were already past the age when diet has its most powerful effect. In China, for example, the dietary pattern observed was present during the entire life of the individual, including his/her childhood.

The second possibility is that the lower ranges of saturated fat intake tested in all these cohort studies were not sufficiently low enough to be protective. The dietary variation from one group to another was not large enough to show a significant difference.

The bottom line is that these studies on adults in Western countries are not very accurate. They follow adults who made only moderate dietary changes later in life, and who were likely past the age when dietary influence can have a pronounced effect on cancer occurrence.

GROWING CELLS ARE MORE SUSCEPTIBLE TO DAMAGING INFLUENCES

The growing body, with its dividing cells, is at greater risk when exposed to all types of negative and toxic influences. In adults, our valuable genetic material (DNA) is wound up in a tight ball, like the rubber bands on the inside of a golf ball. When we are young and cells are replicating and growing, the DNA unwinds, exposing more of its surface. This makes it more susceptible to damage from toxic exposure. According to the U.S. Environmental Protection Agency, infants and toddlers have a ten times greater cancer risk than adults when exposed to gene-damaging chemicals.[12] In a similar manner, an unhealthy diet can do substantially more damage to a young body than to an adult one. The earlier in life, the greater the potential for damage.

For example, breast cancer is associated with high body weight and obesity. Of particular interest is the fact that body weight in the twenty years prior to the time the cancer is diagnosed has not been consistently correlated with increased risk. It is body weight much earlier in life that showed the consistent effect. Some researchers conclude that dieting in later life may be too late.[13]

In one of the largest studies of weight gain and breast cancer ever performed, researchers documented that even modest amounts of weight gain after age eighteen is a strong predictor of cancer later in life. The closer to the teenage years that the weight was put on and the more weight that was gained increased the risk of breast cancer proportionally. Obesity increases the incidence of many common cancers. For example, a carefully designed study that tracked more than one million women for twenty-five years found that women who were heavier and taller as youngsters were 56 percent more likely to develop ovarian cancer.[14] This does not mean that weight gain later in life does not increase cancer risk. It just means that the risk factors are stronger in certain more sensitive age brackets. This is still a realm where much more research needs to be done. One thing we know for sure is that people who maintain a thin or normal weight for their entire lives have much lower cancer rates. We cannot eat in an unrestrained, unhealthful manner in our youth and expect healthful dieting at a later point in life to undo all the damage.

The idea that eating an anti-cancer diet in our childhood is more important in determining cancer risk than waiting to eat healthy as an adult has been tested in animals by Dr. Jerald Silverman of the Comprehensive Cancer Center at Ohio State University with a grant from the American Institute for Cancer Research. He chose to study a strain of mice very susceptible to breast cancer. He put one group on a diet low in fat their entire lives and he switched the other group from a high-fat diet to a healthier low-fat one at different times, some before puberty, some at puberty, and some after puberty. The study showed the same thing we see in human studies: those mice fed the high-fat diet had more cancer and more of the cancer spread to the lung, and the earlier the change to the healthier lower-fat diet, the better the mice fared.

Not just breast cancer, but other cancers demonstrate a similar age-sensitive relationship as well. Colon cancer is associated with obesity, but this association is still weak. The association becomes much stronger if we see it beginning at a younger age. Body weight in adolescents more strongly correlates with colon cancer in adults.[15]

The same is true with ovarian cancer, which shows an even stronger relationship with excessive weight gain in early childhood and even infancy. Weight gain during the first few years of life also implicates the mother's diet during gestation and nursing in the causality of ovarian cancer.[16] Harvard Medical School researchers found that women who reported being overweight by age eighteen were twice as likely to be diagnosed with ovarian cancer later in life.[17] Obviously, what you are fed much earlier in life and the dietary habits you learn through your parents lead to becoming an overweight teenager with higher risks down the road.

CHILDHOOD EXPOSURE HAS THE LARGEST IMPACT ON ADULT HEALTH

The things we are exposed to earlier in life are crucial to our later health. If a nuclear power plant exploded nearby, dousing us all in heavy radiation, it would not cause a significant increase in cancer occurrence for about twenty-five years. For example, the excess risk for breast, prostate, and colon cancer among atomic bomb survivors in Hiroshima and Nagasaki continues to be observed today, and persists throughout the lifetime of the survivors. The largest grouping of the radiation-related cancer deaths for these common cancers occurred in the period from 1986 to 1990, forty to forty-five years after exposure.[18]

We see the same lag time between other events that initiate and promote cancer. The link between low-plant-fiber diets and higher consumption of animal products many years before a cancer finally appears is illustrated by the changing diet in Japan and the growing incidence of colon cancer. The intake of Total Dietary Fiber (TDF) was evaluated from data from the National Nutrition Survey in Japan for forty-one years beginning in 1947. TDF intake decreased rapidly from 27.4 grams per day in 1947 to 15.8 grams in 1963. Fat intake increased rapidly from 18 grams in 1950 to 56.6 grams in 1987. Of significance in this carefully done study was that the increased occurrence of colon cancer had a twenty-three-to-twenty-four-year lag after the heightened consumption of animal products began. Apparently what the Japanese people did twenty-five years earlier had the strongest effect on inducing cancer, not what they ate ten years or even twenty years earlier.[19] Those with the highest consumption of plant fiber in their childhood had the lowest incidence of colon cancer.

Recent studies have also found that eating fruit during childhood had powerful effects to protect against cancer in later life. A sixty-year study of 4,999 participants found that those who consumed more fruit in their childhood (the highest quartile) were 38 percent less likely to develop cancer as adults.[20]

Diets rich in meat and dairy are powerfully implicated as cancer promoters. Processed, pickled, smoked, or barbequed meats are even

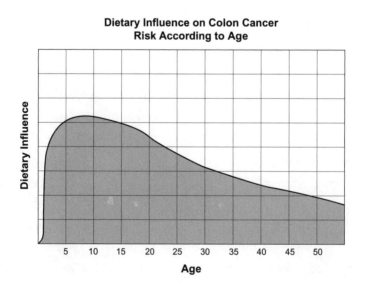

Dietary Influence on Colon Cancer Risk According to Age

more strongly linked to cancer. Separate studies from Europe and the United States found the same results: those who eat meat daily have a three- to four-fold increase incidence of colon, esophageal, and stomach cancers, and the risks are more severe the younger in age people begin these practices.[21]

Nasopharyngeal carcinoma (NPC) is a perfect example of a childhood-induced adult cancer. It occurs predominantly in populations consuming heavily salted products, preserved foods, and hot spices such as hot chili sauce. Salted fish, processed meats, and preserved foods contain nitrites and nitrosomines, a known animal carcinogen. A meticulous study added up the total amount of nitrates and nitrosomines from all dietary sources throughout various ages in the life of 375 cases of nasopharyngeal carcinoma and 327 controls without the disease. They found that the intake of nitrosomines and nitrite as a child was predictive of later cancer, though the consumption of these compounds as an adult was not associated with an increased occurrence of NPC. The intake of green vegetables during childhood was shown to be protective. The study concluded that the risk and incidence of NPC was accounted for by the higher levels of nitrite and nitrosomine compounds consumed during childhood.[22] The growing body, with more rapidly dividing cells, is more sensitive to damage from chemical compounds; the cells become dysplastic (an abnormal, precancerous condition), and over the years turn cancerous. Many years later, the cancer becomes detectable.

FEED THEM SO THEY GROW BIG AND STRONG?

Recent studies are lending powerful support confirming the position that most adult cancers are strongly associated with overeating, eating less fruits and vegetables, and eating more dairy, meats, and processed food during childhood. Many parents enthusiastically strive to overfeed their children with the purpose of achieving excessive growth. While childhood growth and early maturity have been hailed by some as a success of this century, the scientific data questions these common objectives.

Numerous scientific investigations report the relationship between high calorie intake in childhood and cancer. One recent study followed 3,834 subjects for over fifty years, measuring dietary intake in childhood. They collected data on children's diets between 1937 and 1939. This study found a positive association between calories consumed during early life and later mortality from every cancer other than those related to smoking. Each increased energy intake of 1 MJ/day (238 calories) was associated with a 20 percent increased risk of mortality from the most common cancers.[23] Fewer calories consumed during childhood provided protection against all three common cancers (breast, prostate, colon). The researchers concluded that:

> This positive association between childhood energy (caloric) intake and later cancer is consistent with animal evidence linking energy restriction with reduced incidence of cancer and the association between height and human cancer, implying that higher levels of energy intake in childhood increase the risk of later development of cancer. This evidence for long term effect of early diet confirms the importance of optimal nutrition in childhood and suggests that the unfavorable trends seen in the incidence of some cancers may have their origins in early life.

Today our children's caloric consumption is at an all-time high. With all the high-calorie, low-nutrient processed foods, soft drinks, fast foods, pizza, cheese, and butter kids eat today, the girth of America's children is increasing at an alarming rate.[24] This foretells an increase in the cancer epidemic in the future. Little do parents know—their children are eating themselves to death.

Scientific studies have consistently repeated the observation that most common cancers are associated with stimulated growth in childhood, especially growth fueled by a diet heavy in growth-promoting animal products. This protein- and fat-rich diet is enabling today's children to exceed the height predicted by their parental genetics. But children who mature early and grow taller than expected by parental height have been shown to be at higher risk of breast, prostate, colorectal, leukemic, ovarian, and endometrial cancers.[25]

Animal models have displayed this phenomenon for decades.[26] We now have the data to conclude that the same is true for humans. Growth can be equated with aging; slower growth leads to slower aging and longer life. We used to think rapid growth in our children was a beneficial phenomenon. "Drink your milk. It will help you grow big and strong," parents parroted to their children. Over the years, however, scientists have noted that animals that grow faster and mature quicker, die younger. Now we find that drinking "growth-promoting" cow's milk in early childhood may have negative effects. Humans are designed to be raised on human milk in the first few years of life, not cow's milk. Human milk makes for slower growth. Cow's milk is specially designed for baby cows, and it supplies the nutrients to facilitate the rapid growth natural to cows.

Epidemiological studies consistently show low death rates from breast and prostate cancer where dairy consumption is very low.[27] In areas of the world where breast-feeding is routinely continued past the second birthday, the intake of cow's milk products is exceedingly low. It is likely that this combination of more breast milk and a much later introduction of cow's milk explains the results of these studies linking very low intake of dairy to lower incidence of breast and prostate cancer.

The first two years of life are the critical time period during which the immune system matures and develops. During this

two-year period the body relies on immunoglobulins supplied by
the mother's breast milk to offer protection against infectious
agents. As the child's immune system matures and the child is capable of producing his own immunoglobulins, the digestive tract
gradually closes the gaps that allow mother's immunoglobulins to
squeak through. This beautifully designed system assures that the
child gets the added immune protection from his mother's immune
system in proportion to his needs. These needs for the mother's
immunoglobulins decrease gradually as the second birthday is
approached.

These gaps between cells in the immature digestive tract are also
the reason why feeding solid foods to children when they are
young can increase the risk of allergies. The younger the infant begins to eat food, rather than breast milk, the more likely food components, not adequately digested yet, can squeak through the
digestive tract and enter the bloodstream, leading to the development of food allergies.

Milk for humans is made by female humans. Cow's milk is perfectly designed for the rapid growth needs and brain requirements
of cows. Breast milk, with its immunoglobins and brain-supporting
nutrients, is designed to be the perfect food for the developing human. If we expect our children to grow up healthfully we must supply them with the normal requirements of human existence,
requirements that include human milk, real food (not fake food),
and protection from toxic drugs.

Cheese consumption during childhood is a major concern because it takes ten pounds of milk to make one pound of cheese. Besides the bovine growth hormone given to cows, their milk contains
estrogen, progesterone, testosterone, prolactin, and other natural
cow hormones. Cheese not only is richer in saturated fat, but is a
more concentrated source of these hormones. These milk hormones
can exert effects on humans.[28] The more you drink or eat dairy, the
more hormones you get, and cheese consumption magnifies the

negative aspects of cow's milk. Whether it is the hormonal exposure, the high levels of saturated fat, or the growth-promoting effects, any way you look at it, the vastly successful advertising campaign waged on Americans has given milk and cheese an unearned health food status. Science suggests otherwise, and slower growth and a later maturation are favorable to longer life.

More and more studies are emerging that illustrate that rapid growth at an early age shows an even stronger association to cancer than simply being overweight.[29] Being overweight is not typically an early childhood occurrence. Dietary excesses in early childhood and the consumption of growth-promoting foods such as cow's milk, cheese, and meat is marked by acceleration in growth and an earlier attainment of adult height and size. We should want our children to grow slowly. The faster they grow and the faster they reach puberty, the faster they age and the greater the risk of getting a later-life cancer.

Bigness is not a criteria for health. Certainly, eating rich foods and lots of animal foods can help us more easily achieve our potential to become a 200-to-350-pound male human, but is that ideal for health and longevity? It is not. When we look at the longevity of large, overly muscled football linebackers, we find reduced longevity. A research study conducted by the National Institute of Occupational Safety and Health (NIOSH) examined the later life health of 6,848 former NFL players. They found that the largest players, offensive and defensive linemen, had a 50 percent greater risk of heart disease than the general population (which is already at a whopping 40%) and a 3.7 times increased risk of dying from heart disease compared to other (smaller and leaner) football players.[30] NIOSH researcher Dr. Sherry Baron stated, "Clearly the increased body size typical of these positions is contributing to the substantial risk. Anyone considering bulking up to play football should also consider the very real threat of heart disease." Although obesity has been linked to cardiovascular disease in many research studies, the

NIOSH study found the strongest association between body size and death. Players in the largest Body Mass Index (BMI) category had six times greater risk of death than those in the lowest BMI category.

There is a strong association in the scientific literature between body size and death. This does not just mean fat on the body. Muscular athletes with the highest BMI have significant increased risk of a premature death. BMI represents a weight-to-height ratio; the higher the number, the more weight per height. One Swedish study followed former athletes with high muscle mass for at least twenty-two years and found that those with high BMI from excess muscular mass had a risk of dying younger that was as bad as that caused by fat-predominant obesity.[31] The goal for superior health is to be strong, lean, and fit; not to be as big as possible.

Recently researchers analyzed data on more than one million women who were tracked for an average of twenty-five years. Teens with a BMI in the top 15 percent were found to be twice as likely to develop ovarian cancer during the twenty-five-year observation period. The tallest girls in the group had the highest risk, so being both tall and heavy was the most risky; being shorter and thinner was protective.[32]

Avoiding calorie-dense, nutrient-poor food such as sugar, oil, white flour, cheese, butter, and fatty meats and instead substituting vegetables, beans, and fruits helps control excessive consumption of calories. Eliminating empty calories is the only reasonable method for extending lifespan and slowing aging.

Although the first experiments on dietary and calorie manipulations were performed over sixty years ago in rodents, in more recent years these tests have been applied to numerous species and have been conducted in primates since 1987.[33] Monkeys given more nutrients but less calories not only live longer, but have a slower aging process. In much of today's world, parents do the exact opposite of what science has shown to prevent cancer and extend life. We feed our children a high-calorie, low-nutrient diet, instead of a protective, high-nutrient, lower-calorie diet. This forebodes an explosive cancer epidemic in years to come. The World Health Organization predicts that cancer rates will increase alarmingly, by 50 percent by 2020, if nothing is done to stem this trend.[34]

BREAST CANCER CAUSATION IS MULTIFACTORIAL

Worldwide, there is a linear relationship between higher-fat animal products, saturated fat intake, and breast cancer.[35] However, there are areas of the world even today where populations eat predominantly unrefined plant foods in childhood and breast cancer is simply unheard of. Rates of breast cancer deaths (in the 50-to-70 age range) range widely from 3.4 per 100,000 in Gambia to 10 per 100,000 in rural China, 20 per 100,000 in India, 90 per 100,000 in the United States, and 120 per 100,000 in the United Kingdom and Switzerland.[36]

Experimental evidence suggests that the susceptibility of mammary tissue to carcinogenesis is greatest in the childhood and teenage years. The time during breast growth and development is a particularly sensitive period in a woman's life, affecting the later development of breast cancer in adulthood. Teenagers who eat more high-fiber, high-antioxidant foods such as fruits, vegetables, and nuts have less occurrence of benign breast disease, the precursor marker of breast cancer.[37]

Of particular concern is the pattern linking breast cancer to the early age of puberty we are witnessing in modern times. The average age of onset of menstruation in the nineteenth century was seventeen, whereas in the last fifty years in Western industrialized countries, such as the United States, the average age of onset of menstruation is twelve. The overnutrition and heightened exposure to animal products, oils, and saturated fats[38] earlier in life induces a rapid earlier growth and an earlier puberty. Earlier age of puberty increases one's lifetime exposure to estrogens and is associated with a higher incidence of breast cancer years later.

Cohort studies, which follow two groups of children over time, have shown that the higher consumption of produce and protein-rich plant foods such as beans and nuts is associated with a later menarche, and the higher consumption of protein-rich animal foods—meat and dairy—is associated with an earlier menarche and increased occurrence of adult breast cancer.[39]

Early puberty is strongly associated with breast cancer, and the occurrence of breast cancer is three times higher in women who started puberty before age twelve.[40]

A recent intelligently devised study investigated all twin sisters in northern Europe and England where one developed breast cancer and the other did not. The researchers found 400 cases of breast cancer in only one twin occurring before the age of fifty. They concluded that childhood growth before puberty (the twin with cancer was most often taller at age ten) and developing breasts before her cancer-free twin sister was the primary marker of the increased risk.[41]

Another recent study published in the *New England Journal of Medicine* looked at 1,811 sets of twins and reported that for identical twins with cancer, the first twin to reach puberty was five times more likely to develop cancer at an earlier age.[42] The link was even stronger when menstruation began before the age of twelve. Jo Ann Mason, M.D., of Harvard's Brigham and Woman's Hospital said the implications of the study are worrisome given the gradual decline in the age of puberty in the United States and the rise in childhood obesity.

Physicians are seeing more and more girls with precocious sexual development, even before today's average age of twelve, and medical studies confirm that the trend is real and getting worse. How early are our children developing today? At age eight, almost half of black girls and 15 percent of white girls start developing breasts or pubic hair. At age nine, those numbers change to 77 percent of black girls and a third of white girls.[43]

The critical questions, which our nation generally ignores, are how harmful is this and what can be done about it? Obviously, this anomaly in human history where girls mature so young is threatening. We will undoubtedly see breast cancer occurrence continue to climb as today's children reach adulthood. Cancer occurrence has been shown to occur many years after dysplastic changes occur to the breast, and these changes are often visible in teenagers.

It is of particular importance to note the most significant age range where dietary intake most critically affects the age of puberty. A 1999 study published in the *American Journal of Epidemiology* followed children since birth and reported that the girls who consumed more animal products and fewer vegetables between ages one and eight were prone to early maturation and puberty, but the strongest predictor was a diet rich in animal protein before age five.[44]

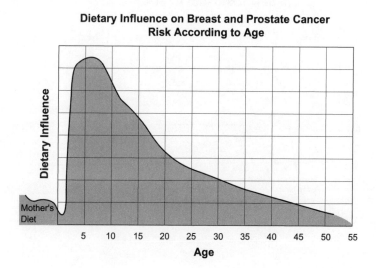

Dietary Influence on Breast and Prostate Cancer Risk According to Age

ESTROGEN, TESTOSTERONE, AND THEIR EFFECTS
ON CHILDREN

Estrogen unquestionably stimulates the development and growth of breast cancer cells. However, it is timing of this exposure that is most crucial and highly complicated. Heightened estrogen exposure at a particular age may increase breast cancer risk, while at another age it does not. These relationships are complex and poorly understood, but one thing we know for sure: girls with early puberty have much higher estrogen levels, and they maintain these significantly higher levels for many years thereafter.[45]

The area under the curve in the graph below reflecting the level of estrogen and testosterone in the bloodstream correlates well with the geographic distribution of breast cancer. Those individuals who develop breast cancer have been found to have higher blood levels of these hormones than those who do not develop breast cancer.[46]

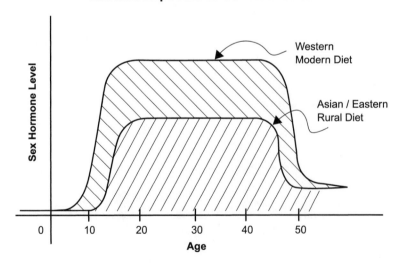

Lifetime Exposure to Sex Hormones

Fat cells produce estrogen, so excess fat on the body during childhood results in more estrogen production. A large volume of high fiber from fruits and vegetables in the gut serves to lower circulating estrogen naturally. The high fiber and the resultant healthy bacteria that colonize the gut of a person consuming a high-produce diet conjugates (binds together) estrogens so they are more readily excreted in the stool. As estrogen cycles into and out of the digestive tract, a person eating more animal products and less high-fiber vegetation reabsorbs more estrogen from the digestive tract, rather than losing more in the stool.

Diet powerfully modulates estrogen levels. One recent study illustrated that eight-to-ten-year-olds, closely followed with dietary intervention for seven years, dramatically lowered their estrogen levels compared to a control group without dietary modification.[47] Clearly, changing the diet of our children after the age of eight is not futile. It will lower the risk of developing cancer, even when the most sensitive years affecting growth and age of puberty have passed. The good news is that we are not helpless after childhood to reduce the risk.

One recent study published in the *Journal of the National Cancer Institute* followed almost 100,000 women between the ages of 26 and 46 and found that the younger the woman was, the greater the effect diet had on later breast cancer incidence. These researchers noted that the consumption of animal fat from predominantly dairy foods and meat was the culprit most closely associated with the occurrence of breast cancer.[48] This study showed a clear-cut, but not large, increase in risk in the women with higher consumption of saturated fat. This study illustrates that making important changes early in adult life can still lower risks of breast cancer. It is never too late to lessen anyone's risk. While our childhood diet is an important factor in the cancer causation equation, it does not mean we are thereafter helpless to prevent cancer. The reason the study referenced above does not show such a large increased risk from the consumption of high-saturated-fat foods is because even in your late twenties and thirties, it is somewhat late to offer the strongest protective shield against cancer that one would have achieved if dramatic dietary improvements were started early in life and maintained. As we get older, the opportunity to *dramatically* lower risk diminishes. **Little changes in childhood make a difference; big changes in adulthood are needed to compensate for little nutritional mistakes in childhood.**

Having children and breast-feeding those children as long as possible, combined with a lifestyle that includes good nutrition and exercise, can also reduce risk and help the early pathological changes in the breast revert back to normal.[49]

SECRET CHEMICALS IN OUR FOOD

The Institute of Medicine of the National Academy of Science released a public report in June 2003, warning the public about the cancer risk from consuming food containing dioxin and other polychlorobiphenyls (PCBs). The Institute of Medicine advises the federal government on medical matters and appoints experts to research and produce these reports. The report concluded with the statement:

The most direct way for an individual or a population to reduce dietary intake of dioxins is to reduce their consumption of dietary fat, especially from animal sources that are known to contain higher levels of these compounds.

This report from the National Academy of Science came out only one day after the Environmental Protection Agency reported that the amount of dioxin released into the environment by industry increased to 328 pounds in 2001, up from 220 pounds the year earlier. The EPA added that 6.16 billion pounds of toxic chemicals were released into the environment in 2001.

The EPA explained that these compounds persist in the environment and build up in the bodies of farm animals that eat contaminated feed or grass. While many of these toxic chemical compounds are resistant to degradation in the natural environment, they dissolve readily in oil and thus accumulate in the fatty tissues of fish, birds, and mammals. Humans are exposed predominantly by eating contaminated animal products. Every time an animal is exposed to a tiny bit of these toxic chemicals, it remains in the animal's body for life, only released when the animal is eaten by humans, through fatty animal products such as meat, cheese, and full-fat milk.[50] Animal products tested to be exceptionally high in these harmful compounds are catfish, lobster, mollusks, cheese, butter, and ice cream.[51]

Unborn children and breast-feeding infants are especially vulnerable to the harmful effects of these chemicals. These chemicals are linked to a broad range of diseases, including behavioral disorders, thyroid dysfunction, endometriosis, and cancer.[52] Since these chemicals are stored in the fatty tissues of animals and in our fat stores, too (because we are animals as well), a woman has to begin eating more carefully before she gets pregnant to prevent harmful exposure to the developing fetus.

The health of children is not merely the result of what they have been fed as youngsters, but is strongly influenced by a mother's diet and what she consumed and stored in her fat-supply years before her child is conceived. The National Academy of Science gave a clear public warning against eating a diet rich in animal fats, especially fatty fish and shellfish. Again, a plant-based diet containing healthy fat from avocados, raw nuts, and seeds, with much less or no animal fats, is revealed as a powerful weapon to beat the modern cancer epidemic.

Nursing also helps protect against breast cancer. During lactation, the secretion of estrogens in a woman's body falls to virtually nil, and continuing to breast-feed for a prolonged period has a significant effect on resetting her estrogen to a lower lever thereafter.[53] Maximum protection is achieved after breast-feeding for approximately two years, which corresponds with the baby's immunologic development, maximizing protection against disease for the baby as well. So breast-feeding plays a role in protecting both the baby and the mother from developing cancer.

The American Cancer Society reports that approximately 200,000 new cases of breast cancer were diagnosed in the United States in 2002 and about 40,000 breast cancer deaths occurred.[54] Despite extensive research and the establishment of breast cancer screening programs, these statistics have changed little in the past four decades. We must attack this disease at its roots and stop so much unnecessary suffering and death.

PROSTATE CANCER: A GROWING DISEASE IN MEN

The studies examining the link between obesity, body size, and prostate cancer have focused on adult Body Mass Index (BMI). The results of these studies have not been conclusive; some studies have found a direct relationship and others have not.[55] When looking carefully at tallness versus obesity, there is an apparent link between prostate cancer and height, but not with obesity. This is probably because extra fat on the body results in a higher estrogen/progesterone ratio, and it is the higher testosterone/estrogen ratio that promotes prostate cancer. Therefore, the earlier attainment of adult height is more closely related to prostate cancer risk, not merely being overweight. Men over seventy-one inches tall were observed to have a 32 percent increased risk of prostate cancer. The conclusion is that the dietary style that is the most growth-promoting also promotes a higher level of testosterone in childhood that is linked to later-life prostate cancer.[56]

It takes at least one generation for men in immigrant families coming to America to assume the cancer risks of their host country, suggesting the importance of early-life factors.[57] Similar to early puberty in females, earlier attainment of adult height and early onset of beard growth in males is a marker of increased risk of prostate cancer.[58] Men's diets as toddlers and children most powerfully affect the age when they mature and develop facial hair. The prostate gland is essentially a dormant organ until puberty (much like the female breast), when heightened testosterone levels stimulate its development.

The data on prostate cancer causation points to higher testosterone levels beginning at an earlier age in childhood and throughout puberty as having a strong effect on later occurrence and aggressiveness of prostate cancer.[59] Furthermore, studies demonstrate that prostate intraepithelial neoplasia, a cancer precursor lesion, is already common in men in their twenties and thirties, suggesting that the process of carcinogenesis begins early.[60]

Prostate cancer is the male version of breast cancer. The genetic predisposition is illustrated by the fact that families with a strong history of breast cancer have an increased risk of prostate cancer in their male offspring and vice versa. So the early nutritional environment we grow our children in creates the favorable soil to fuel the breast cancer and prostate cancer epidemics. The same dietary factors that heighten estrogen levels in females raise testosterone levels in males.

When the death rates for prostate and testicular cancer were examined in forty-two countries and correlated with dietary practices in a carefully designed study, they found that cheese consumption was most closely linked with the incidence of testicular cancer for ages twenty to thirty-nine, and milk was the most closely associated with prostate cancer of all foods.[61] Meat, coffee, and animal fats also showed a positive correlation.

ARE PESTICIDES A SERIOUS HEALTH HAZARD?

Acute lymphoblastic leukemia is up 10.7 percent over the last twenty years. Brain cancer is up 30 percent; osteogenic sarcoma, a type of bone cancer, is up 50 percent; and testicular cancer is up 60 percent in men under thirty. No one can tell us why. Scientific studies provide clues that are difficult to ignore:

- Children whose parents work with pesticides are more likely to suffer leukemia, brain cancer, and other afflictions.

- Studies show that childhood leukemia is related to increased pesticide use around the house.

- Nine studies reviewed by the National Cancer Institute showed a correlation between pesticide exposure and brain cancer.

- Exposure to weed killers in childhood increases asthma risk by more than fourfold.

All the dangers stated above are not the result of eating pesticide-treated produce. This clear link between pesticides and cancer is a result of chemical use around the home and farm.[62] Clearly, it is not logical to eat organic food to avoid pesticide residue and then spray our homes with carcinogenic insecticides and weed killers used liberally in and around homes, interior plants, lawns, gardens, and even schools.

Because young children are the ones most susceptible to toxic exposures, the National Academy of Science has issued warnings and position papers stating that exposure to pesticides in early life can increase cancer rates down the road as well as increasing the occurrence of mental and immune system disorders.[63]

We must be careful not to expose our children to chemical cleaners, insecticides, and weed killers on our lawns. Chemicals used in pressure-treated wood used to build lawn furniture, decks, fences, and swing sets have also been shown to place children at risk. When young children are around, we must be vigilant to maintain a chemical-free environment.

The Environmental Protection Agency reports that the majority of pesticides now in use are probable or possible cancer causers. Studies of farm workers who work with pesticides suggest a link between pesticide use and brain cancer, Parkinson's disease, multiple myloma, leukemia, lymphoma, and cancers of the stomach, prostate, and testes.[64] But the question remains, does the low level of pesticides remaining on our food present much of a danger?

Some scientists argue that the extremely low level of pesticide residue remaining on produce is insignificant and that there are naturally occurring toxins in all natural foods that are more significant. The large amount of studies performed on the typical pesticide-treated produce have demonstrated that consumption of produce, whether organic or not, is related to lower rates of cancer and disease protection, not higher rates. Certainly, it is better to eat fruits and vegetables grown and harvested using pesticides than not eating them at all. The health benefits of eating phytochemical-rich produce greatly outweigh any risk pesticide residues might pose.

It has been shown that women with higher levels of pesticides in their bloodstream have a higher risk of breast cancer.[65] However, the pesticide shown in these studies to be connected to cancer was DDT, which is no longer used in food production and was banned by the U.S. government in 1972. The problem is that DDT is still in the environment and finds its way back into our food supply, predominately via shellfish and fish consumption. So purchasing organic fruits and vegetables will not lower our exposure to DDT if we are eating fish and shellfish regularly.

Keep in mind, there is a significantly larger exposure to toxic chemicals in animal products compared to plant foods. By eating lower on the food chain and reducing our intake of animal products, one automatically reduces exposure to toxic chemicals. Plants have the least fat-soluble pollutants, animals that eat plants have more, and animals that eat animals have the highest levels of these toxic compounds. Fish that eat smaller fish will store the toxic compounds from every fish it ever ate, including all the fish eaten by the fish it just made a meal of. It is important to avoid lobster, shellfish, catfish, and predator fish such as tuna, bluefish, striped bass, shark, and swordfish, where toxins such as PCB, DDT, dioxin, and mercury are likely to build up due to the compounding effects of eating lots of smaller fish. One gets larger doses of more toxic compounds from these contaminated animal products than would be possible to take in from produce.

Organic food is certainly your best bet, to further limit exposure to toxic chemicals. No one knows for sure how much risk exists from the pesticide residue on produce, but here's what we do know: the younger you are, the more your cells are susceptible to damage from toxins. It seems wise to try to feed our young children organic food whenever possible.

Of course, wash your vegetables and fruit with water and when possible, use a drop of dishwashing detergent and then rinse well to remove all detergent residues for a little more efficient cleaning. Specialty pesticide removal products have not clearly demonstrated any more effectiveness than mild soap and water.

Besides the heightened exposure to chemicals and pesticides from animal products, the most hazardous pesticides are used on some plant foods responsible for the majority of the plant-food-related

LESSEN YOUR EXPOSURE TO PESTICIDES

After peeling and discarding the skin of bananas, mangoes, oranges, pineapples, and melons, wash your hands with soap before touching, serving, or eating them.

Peel and discard skin of potatoes and carrots, unless organic.

Peel cucumbers, apples, peaches, and pears, unless organic.

Remove and discard outer leaves of cabbage and lettuce.

Trim all fat and skin from poultry or other animal foods.

Avoid eating fruits imported from other countries, unless they have skins that can be removed and discarded.

Do not eat nonorganic strawberries or feed them to children. Use frozen organic when fresh organic are not available or too expensive.

dietary risk. These foods with the most pesticide residue are: strawberries, peaches, raspberries, blackberries, grapes, cherries, apples, and celery. Imported produce is also more likely to contain higher levels of pesticides.[66]

There is another reason to feed our children organic food when possible. Organic food usually has more nutrients than conventional.[67] One study performed at the University of California at Davis found that foods grown organically had higher amounts of flavonoids, which have protective effects against both heart disease and cancer. The researchers found that flavonoids were more than 50 percent higher in organic corn and strawberries. They theorized that when the plants are forced to deal with the stress of insects, they produce more of these compounds, which are beneficial to humans.[68] Overall, organic foods taste better, and organic agriculture protects farmers and our environment.

HEART DISEASE STARTS YOUNG, TOO

There is considerable evidence that the lipoprotein abnormalities (high LDL and low HDL) that are linked to heart attack deaths in adulthood begin to develop in early childhood and that higher cholesterol levels eventually get "set" by early food habits.[69] What we eat during our childhood affects our lifetime cholesterol levels. For many, changing the diet to a plant-based, low-saturated-fat diet in later life does not result in the favorable cholesterol levels that would have been seen if the dietary improvements were started much earlier in life.

As a result of the heart-unfriendly diet, blood vessel damage begins early. Not only does the development of coronary athero-sclerosis develop in childhood, but the earlier development of ath-erosclerosis and higher serum cholesterol levels in childhood result in a significantly higher risk of premature sudden death relatively early in life. Sometimes the effects of childhood dietary abuses can be seen relatively early, with premature death or a heart attack at a young age.

When we study people who died young of coronary artery disease, we find that the highest risk of an earlier death occurs in those who were above average weight in childhood.[70] Findings from the famous Bogalusa Heart Study show that a high saturated fat intake early in life is strongly predictive of later heart disease burden and that higher blood pressure in childhood and adoles-cence is powerfully predictive of cardiovascular death in adult-hood.[71]

A low-fiber, high-saturated-fat diet with lots of animal products, dairy fat, white flour, and sugar creates a heart attack–prone person with high cholesterol levels. The anti-cancer lifestyle, a healthy diet style for the entire family, started early in life, will have the added benefit of making it easier for children to become heart

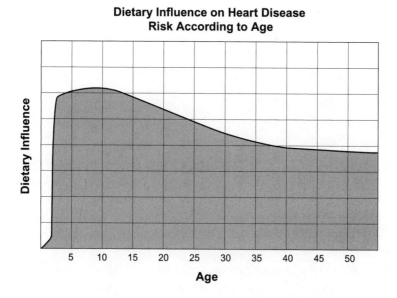

attack–proof. A diet high in plant fiber shows a protective effect against developing high cholesterol, obesity, and elevated insulin levels. Eating more of the natural high-fiber plant food in childhood has a powerful protective effect on preventing later-life heart problems, even for those with a strong family history of heart disease.[72] For those whose family genetically predisposes them to heart disease, early-life dietary excellence can make the difference between a long life free of heart disease and a heart attack in one's forties or fifties.

The new recommendations developed by the American Heart Association's Council on Cardiovascular Disease in the Young acknowledge that heart disease starts early in life and that the eating habits and food preferences that are continued into adulthood are more difficult to change. They advise the entire family to limit salt and saturated fat. This is an important message for our society to understand. Heart disease may be preventable and reversible with nutritional excellence in adulthood, but in most cases, people do too little too late and suffer the tragic consequences—40 percent of the American population is still dying of heart disease.

Heart disease as a pediatric disease best treated by physicians with the ability to intercede during childhood is an issue that has been discussed by researchers in this field for almost twenty years. At a 1986 heart disease symposium, Roger Williams, M.D., the director of Cardiovascular Genetic Research and professor of medicine at the University of Utah School of Medicine, explained that the best way to prevent heart disease in genetically prone patients is to intervene in childhood. He reported, when looking at those genetically predisposed to heart disease, that the only way to strongly protect against a sudden heart attack death at a comparatively young age is to intervene in their youth.[73] He also said that telling patients and their families to "watch fat" is insufficient.

Scientific literature has continued to strongly support the view that coronary artery disease leading to heart attacks is an avoidable event, even for those with a strong family history. It is the high nutritional quality of the diet, with more fruits, vegetables, beans, and healthy fats from raw nuts and seeds that offers the type of protection that is really effective.

WHAT WE DO KNOW CAN HELP OUR CHILDREN

We must be responsible for our health and the health of our children. We parents have a huge responsibility and can help guide and shape our offspring into healthy and happy adults, or, through abuse, neglect, ignorance, and even convenience, we can damage their future. We know with certainty that the foods we feed our kids during childhood play a large role in dictating their future health.

We know that children have sensitive vulnerabilities that are quite distinct from adults. Their exposure to chemicals in our environment is more potentially damaging than the same exposure at a later age. It is important to realize that the diet a woman eats during her pregnancy and even before her pregnancy effects the adult health of her future offspring. For example, a recent study shows a strong association in children who develop brain tumors with the mother's consumption of hot dogs during pregnancy.[74] Scientific evidence suggests that cigarette smoking during pregnancy is associated with testicular cancer in sons thirty-five to fifty years later.[75] We may get away with risky behaviors when we imbibe in our later years, but when we gamble with our children, the stakes are much higher and the damage more profound.

Health is a complicated issue. All the contributory causes of cancer and other diseases are not presently known. A variety of external factors interact with genetics to initiate and propagate the process of carcinogenesis. Multiple factors come into play to induce damage leading to cancer. Nevertheless, the preponderance of evidence demonstrates that superior nutrition can almost always overwhelm a family history of cancer. The vast majority of cancers are still avoidable.

In present-day society, we are experiencing a modern form of malnutrition never before known in human history. Unfortunately, our population is making food choices for themselves and their children virtually unaware of the risks they are taking. At least know the level of the water in the deep end before you jump blindly in.

While I cannot overemphasize the importance of childhood nutrition, nutritional excellence in later life can have profound effects at reducing the risk of life-threatening disease and cancer, as well as provide positive effects on survival and well-being throughout life. I have even observed patients with cancer adopt programs of nutritional excellence and demonstrate recovery. This book is not written to encourage anyone to think that they cannot improve their diet and reduce the probability of getting cancer at any age, or increase your chances for survival or recovery if you have cancer. Sooner is better, but eating well at any age can lead to overall health.

four

Feeding Your Family for Superior Health

The time to begin paying attention to a child's health is long before birth. Even the mother's diet twelve months before conception can influence the child's future health. It is important to eat healthfully prior to conception as well as once pregnancy has begun. Proper nutrition and good health habits are more important than ever during pregnancy and can help in maintaining good health for both mother and baby.

PRECAUTIONS TO TAKE WHEN PREGNANT OR NURSING

The developing baby inside you is sensitive to the effects of toxins, more so than at any other time in its life. It is never too early to start protecting yourself and your unborn child.

Clearly, there are a lot of dangerous habits to avoid before pregnancy, and there are also a lot of fears women have that are not founded in science or logic.

The real concerns are not microwave ovens, cell phones, and hair dryers. The things we know to be really risky for you and your unborn children are:

Caffeine

Nicotine, including secondhand smoke

Alcohol

Medications, both over-the-counter and prescription drugs

Herbs and high-dose supplements, vitamin A

Fish, mollusks and shellfish, sushi (raw fish)

Hot tubs and saunas

Radiation

Household cleaner, paint thinners

Cat litter (because of an infectious disease called toxoplasmosis caused by a parasite found in cat feces)

Raw milk and cheese

Soft cheeses and blue-veined cheeses such as feta, Roquefort, and Brie

Artificial colors, nitrates, and MSG

Deli meats, luncheon meats, hot dogs, and undercooked meats

When a pregnant women uses drugs, even aspirin, she and her unborn child can face serious health problems. Also, just because something is natural or purchased in a health food store does not mean it is safe. Herbal remedies work because of their medicinal properties from naturally occurring toxins; they are not health food. I also advise against dyeing your hair during pregnancy.

I advise pregnant women to completely avoid seafood products; it is just too difficult to know what pollution lies within. Shellfish and mollusks are particularly risky.

Toxoplasmosis and listeria are two infectious agents recognized to be dangerous to your unborn child. If you have a cat, only change the litter wearing disposable gloves to reduce the risk of contracting toxoplasmosis. By avoiding raw dairy products, soft cheeses, and undercooked meats, you can reduce the risk of contacting listeria.

Caffeine has been a controversial topic for decades. Evidence clearly concludes that heavy coffee drinkers have an increased risk of miscarriage and low birth weight infants, but the evidence is not clear for moderate users of caffeine.[1] Nevertheless, it is wise to stay away from as many potentially harmful substances as possible. The bottom line, if in doubt, don't do it.

The first year of life is a critical year that sets the stage for your child's healthy body and mind. Exposure to DHA-rich breast milk while the brain is rapidly growing assures that your child will develop his full intelligence potential. To supplement her healthy diet, Mom should be taking a multivitamin plus a daily DHA supplement containing approximately 200 mg of DHA, to assure adequate DHA content in her breast milk. Even after food is introduced, continued breast-feeding is important and necessary past the first birthday for maximum disease resistance, immune function, and brain development.

The avoidance of exposure to chemicals and potential allergens is important during this sensitive stage. Food additives, pesticides, household cleaners, insecticides, and antibiotics should all be scrupulously avoided, as there is an increased sensitivity to their damaging influences in the first year of life.

Exposure to dairy proteins from cow's milk has also shown long-term negative consequences when used very young in life. Delaying the feeding of all food except breast milk until six months is important, and the foods you choose to begin with at six months are important, too.

Most authorities are in agreement today that exclusive breastfeeding is the ideal way to feed infants in the first six months of life. As the digestive tract matures during the first year of life, the spaces between the cells that allow the mother's immunoglobins to be absorbed gradually get tighter, reducing the potential for food allergies.

INTRODUCING YOUR CHILD TO SOLID FOODS

After six months, foods should be introduced gradually, one by one, with the introduction of one new food every two days so the parents can watch for signs of food allergies or sensitivity to a particular food such as a skin rash or digestive discomfort. If you have a strong family history of allergies, the careful recommendations below should be modified somewhat to delay introduction of potentially allergic foods (such as nuts, dairy, soy, corn, wheat, and eggs) even further and to extend the time of exclusive breastfeeding.

SUGGESTED FOODS FOR THE
SIX-TO-NINE-MONTH OLD

I recommend that your baby's first food be banana mashed with breast milk, or organic brown rice cereal made especially for babies mixed with pure water and breast milk. The next week, add some avocado mashed in with a banana. Continue to add new foods gradually over the next few months, utilizing peeled, pureed fresh fruit such as apples, pears, peaches, or papayas. Alternate the fruit feedings with vegetables cooked in a pressure cooker or steamed and then pureed. A hand baby mill is an easy and convenient way to puree cooked vegetables. Commercial organic baby food is a convenient way to serve green peas, peas, carrots, squash, zucchini, string beans, and others. They are convenient when traveling, too, but it is also simple to make your own steamed or pressure-cooked vegetables and then blend them with the remaining liquid in the pressure cooker to make your own mushy veggies. I also suggest steamed asparagus or artichoke hearts mixed with a little sweet potato as an early food.

FOODS TO AVOID IN INFANCY

Do not feed babies anything with added salt, sugar, or honey. Only organic fruits and vegetables and organic baby food should be used. To reduce the chance of developing allergies, delay feeding strawberries and citrus fruits until twelve months of age, and hold off on ground nuts and nut butters until nine months of age. Of course, children should not be given whole nuts until the age of two and a half because of a choking hazard, but raw nut butters and food made with ground raw nuts are fine after nine months of age. Avoid peanuts and peanut butter until the age of two, because they have such a strong potential for food allergy.

Raw nuts and seeds are an excellent source of protein, the healthiest type of fat, and are loaded with minerals and vitamins. Grind up sunflower seeds, almonds, and walnuts and store these ground nuts in the freezer to add to vegetables and fruit dishes for your child after nine months of age.

SUGGESTED FOODS FOR THE NINE-TO-TWELVE-MONTH OLD

By nine months, most children are eating an assortment of healthy food, and at this time they should be introduced to a larger variety in their diet. All steamed and pureed fruits and vegetables are at your disposal, especially peas, corn, carrots, string beans, asparagus, squash, and sweet and white potatoes.

English peas, removed from the pod, can be fed raw after pureeing them in a baby mill. This is a great way to get raw greens into your baby. You can mix some of the pureed raw peas into other foods, too. Raw nuts, especially almonds, sunflower seeds, walnuts, and cashews, can be ground into a powder or made into butters. These ground nuts can be mashed in with a banana or other fruit or with the pureed vegetables. You can also add other grains besides rice, such as steel-cut oats, millet, or quinoa, which you can stew with water and then blend until smooth. Add a little mashed banana, too, and your child will love these nutritious grains.

Any of these foods can be diluted with breast milk. Never add cow's milk or butter. If breast milk is not an option, use baby formula.

Don't be alarmed if you see the food colors in your child's stool; if it is orange from the carrots or green from the peas, that is normal. Do not feed your infants and toddlers fruit juice because

IMPORTANT FOODS TO AVOID (AT LEAST) UNTIL THE FIRST BIRTHDAY

Eggs, fish and other seafood, meat, cow's milk, cheese, butter, oils, wheat, strawberries, oranges, grapefruits, fruit juice, sweeteners, honey, peanuts, and processed foods with additives or salt.

those extra calories will lessen their appetite to eat whole foods, and you want to develop a consistent eating pattern.

AFTER TWELVE MONTHS OF AGE

After the first birthday is a good time to begin feeding vegetable/bean soups that have been made for the rest of the family; just blend them to break up the beans and thicken the soup. After the age of two, you can just let them chew the beans like the rest of the family.

I strongly recommend that breast-feeding be continued to at least eighteen months and preferably two years or longer. After a year, they are eating enough food, so the frequency of breast-feeding diminishes greatly. Many moms find that three to four times per day is all the little ones request at this age. As they get older, two to three nursings per day can be enough to give them benefit after eighteen months of age. If not continuing to breast-feed until eighteen months of age, use formula, not soy milk or cow's milk.

Each baby formula is different from its competitors, but none of them comes close to duplicating the real thing. Human milk is the food best designed for baby humans. No infant formula can duplicate human milk. Human milk contains living cells, hormones, active enzymes, immunoglobulins, and compounds with unique structures that cannot be replicated. Don't forget, human milk is the preferred feeding for all infants, and it is nature's design that this be part of the normal human diet in the first few years of life, not the first few months of life. Informed parents know that if children are to maximize their intellectual and health potential, they must be breast-fed.

Breast-feeding should be continued as long as possible to maximize the benefits of reducing cancer incidence for both the baby and the nursing mother. Prolonged breast-feeding reduces the risk of breast cancer. The American Academy of Pediatrics (AAP) supports the introduction of whole cow's milk after one year of age. I do not. Gastroesophageal reflux, iron deficiency, and calcium and sodium excess may be created by feeding cow's milk to our infants and toddlers.[2] This is not the only reason, however, for not starting cow's milk at age one. Your child's continued intake of the DHA that he would have received from continued breast-feeding is important.

Since formulas with added DHA modeled after breast milk are now available. If the child cannot be breast-fed until at least the age of two, I recommend that between twelve and eighteen months a DHA-supplemented cow's milk formula be utilized. A DHA-supplemented soy milk formula may be substituted for the cow's milk–based formula, but the cow's milk–based formula is preferred, as it contains significantly less aluminum compared to soy-based formulas. Then, after eighteen months, it can slowly be decreased, as a mixture of soy and nut milk (and even some cow's milk) can be used.

Early introduction of cow's milk increases the chance of developing childhood diabetes and can promote that early-in-life growth spurt linked to later life cancers. Your child does not need cow's milk to be healthy, but if used at all, it is very important not to start it before the age of eighteen months. I strongly recommend that cow's milk NOT be utilized as the exclusive drink of babies and toddlers. If you choose to use cow's milk, have the child use an assortment of healthy drinks, utilizing soy, nut, *and* cow's or goat's milk, so that an overdependency on cow's milk is prevented and more nutritional diversity is fostered.

In spite of all the information available about the crucial importance of breast-feeding, only 16 percent of infants in the United States are breast-fed at one year of age. Cow's milk, fruit juice, and French fries are still commonly given to infants before the first birthday.[3] The first two years of life are an opportunity to build a disease-resistant child and to have that child develop healthy eating habits that can last a lifetime. I think if parents realized how important breast-feeding was for the future health of their child, a much higher percentage would breast-feed longer. If there is an insurmountable reason why breast-feeding can't be done, choose a formula that best resembles human milk. Some of the newer formulas have improved designs with DHA added and modified proteins that are nonallergenic.

I do not recommend rice milks for infants and toddlers. The rice-based milks are too sweet and too low in protein and fat. Instead, you can supplement breast milk with a mixture of soy milk, water, almonds, sunflower seeds, and a very small amount of dates for sweetener, and this mixture can be utilized as a drink to supplement the formula-fed baby during the twelve-to-eighteen-month period as formula is gradually phased out. You can blend raw blanched almonds and other nuts and seeds with unsweetened soy milk and a little water until creamy thick milk is made in a Vita-Mix or other high-powered blender for a more nutritional balanced product than soy milk alone.

Babies under the age of two need adequate fat in their diet. As the volume of breast milk decreases in quantity after nine to twelve months, add avocados, tofu, and nut butters (not cheese and butter) to assure they meet their fat requirements. Tofu made into little tasty "cheesecakes" by mashing the firm tofu with mushy dates and ground almonds is loved by kids, too. You can even mix in vegetables such as frozen peas.

REFORMING THE PICKY EATER

Children are not responsible for their poor food choices—their parents are. Excluding those children with chronic illnesses or severe emotional disorders, a nutritionally poor diet is predominantly the result of misinformed parents and incorrect dietary choices. Before you become disheartened, it is important to understand that most children in today's food environment of processed foods, especially from ages two to seven, are picky eaters.

It is not uncommon or abnormal for a child to prefer a narrow range of foods at this age. It is also not unusual for parents to be in an ongoing battle to coax their child to eat in a manner they feel is appropriate. Fortunately, it is possible to put an end to the food wars and solve the problem of how to get your child to eat a healthful diet.

In my practice, it is common for me to see a parent whose child only eats macaroni and cheese, french fries, chicken nuggets, pizza, and cold cereal with milk. Parents routinely tell me, "Johnny won't eat any fruits or vegetables!" Incredible as it seems, high-calorie, trans-fat-filled french fries are the most common vegetable eaten by young children today. Twenty-five percent of children eat fast food french fries daily.

The Petersons brought their three-year-old son, Joshua, to see me because his prior physician had prescribed twelve separate antibiotic prescriptions for recurrent ear infections in less than nine months. Most often, within a few weeks of stopping the antibiotic, he was sick again with another illnesses. The latest advice from their pediatrician was to put Joshua on a low dose of antibiotics continuously to help reduce the incidence of these infections. I explained to them that for Joshua to stay well and not require antibiotics, he had to adopt a dietary program of superior nutrition. They laughed.

The Petersons didn't need me to tell them that Joshua's diet was inadequate. They clearly knew it. They did not think it was possible to get Joshua to eat healthy food. They were wrong. They followed my advice for reforming the picky eater and when they returned to my office one month later, they proudly reported to me that he was eating a diet of all healthy food. Importantly, they accomplished this without difficulty. We stopped his antibiotics, and he proceeded through that winter without any further ear infections.

When a family first brings their chronically ill child in to see me, I insist that the entire family come—both parents and all siblings—so that we can devise a new eating plan for the entire family. The focus is never solely on the ill child. For the ill child to recover, the crucial first step is for the entire family to make a recovery from their less than optimal diet style.

When the Petersons insisted, "Josh won't eat fruits or vegetables," I explained to them that all children would eat healthfully if shipwrecked. True hunger is difficult to deny. If faced with limited options, they will gleefully eat whatever food is available, without intellectual gymnastics to get them to.

It is not necessary to coax them to eat or to eat healthfully. In fact, battling about food with your child is counterproductive. The trick is to adhere to this one most important rule: only permit healthy food in your home. Children will eat whatever is available. They will not starve themselves to death; they adapt easily and learn relatively quickly to like the food that is offered.

When Mrs. Tenenbaum brought her five-year-old son, Billy, to see me, she insisted that he would only eat chocolate chip cookies, pretzels, salted popcorn, and french fries and would starve to death if not given them. I couldn't believe it. The pediatric ear specialist had placed tubes in Billy's ears for recurrent ear infections; it helped little, and now Billy had chronic sinus infections. None of Billy's prior physicians discussed diet with Mrs. Tenenbaum.

I explained to Mrs. Tenenbaum that if I took her son home with me for a few weeks, where cookies and pretzels would not be present, he would not starve to death. She disagreed. She believed Billy had to be given what he wanted or he would not eat. I finally convinced her that if she removed all the unhealthy food from her refrigerator and cupboard and instead stocked up with raw nuts, fresh fruit, corn, sweet potatoes, peas, and fresh fruit, Billy would have no choice but to try some other food to relieve his hunger. Mrs. Tenenbaum agreed to give this a try.

Billy was distressed for the next twenty-four hours and he did not eat. He complained and threw a tantrum. His mom, frantic and unhappy with my advice, phoned me. I convinced her to stick with it a little longer. Billy eventually tried one or two healthy foods that were available, starting with an entire banana and a fresh corn on the cob. He hadn't touched these foods since he was in diapers. Of course, Billy's mom was still nervous that he was eating so little, but he ate enough food to maintain his weight. Within a few weeks he was consuming larger amounts of food, and within a short time, he was consuming the same number of calories as he had before, only now he was eating a healthy diet. Billy and his mom became great examples and advocates of my program; Billy is no longer sick all the time and has actually learned to appreciate a wide variety of healthy food.

FOOD PREFERENCES ARE FORMED BY ONE'S FOOD ENVIRONMENT

Researchers studying children's food choices have found that the earlier in life the food is introduced, the more likely it will be favored. Parents have been shown to give up too easily when offering healthy food to their children. Keep offering the same food, even if your child rejects it. With persistence, it is likely they will eventually try it and even like it. One study showed that about 75 percent of parents gave up after five tries, while the research showed it took eight to fifteen times for children to accept a new food as familiar. Positive reinforcement, praise, and demonstration of family taste preference (showing your child how much you like it over and over) works better than forcing the child to eat it, and is better than bribing the child. Once the child does give it a shot, tasting the food again and again encourages an eventual favorable taste response.

Taste is a learned phenomenon—both children and adults like the foods they were raised on the best. What is most compelling is that a study shows that even the foods that mothers eat while pregnant and nursing affect what their toddlers will prefer.[4] The message is clear: children raised in an environment of natural foods will more likely continue healthful practices as they grow. Scientific investigations illustrate that children most often take on the eating habits of their parents.[5] Research also indicates that adults who consume lots of fruits and vegetables are those who consumed lots of these foods during childhood.

What has been shown *not to work* is for parents to eat one way and force their children to eat a different way. In fact, parents who force dietary restraint on their children while they themselves eat unrestrainedly were shown to have an adverse effect that fostered the development of body fat on their children.[6]

In short, parents need to eat the diet they would like their child's diet to become. In a study done at Penn State University, researchers found that five-year-olds who ate the most fruits and vegetables had parents who did the same.[7] These researchers concluded, "By eating fruits and vegetables themselves, parents can start a lifetime of cancer-fighting food habits."

The avoidance of fruits and vegetables seen in older children, adolescents, and adults originates in life experiences between six months and three years of age. Early and repeated exposure to a variety of fruits and vegetables has shown to increase liking for them later. Because toddlers have small stomachs and may choose to eat less at mealtimes, they should have access to snacks. Unfortunately, the most common snacks for toddlers are cookies, crackers, chips, milk, and fruit drinks (not juice). A snack can and should be real food like fruit, vegetables, bean and nut dips, wholesome soups, and raw nuts.

The amount of calories children require varies greatly based on age, growth stage, and activity level. Most toddlers eat about 1,000 calories a day and most teenagers eat more than 2,300 calories. Some athletically involved teenagers may require more than 4,000 calories a day. Consuming the right amount of food to match their growth and activity needs happens naturally and without effort.

DON'T COERCE CHILDREN TO EAT

Repeat after me: "I will not be concerned with the number of calories consumed by my child." Remember, it is the internal messages from the brain of your child, finely tuned by metabolic messages, that determine hunger. When there is a true physiologic need for calories and when they are truly hungry, they will eat. You may be able to determine what they eat by what is offered or available in your home environment, but you have almost no ability to force your children to consume more food than their own internal drives tell them they need.

It is especially difficult to get a baby or toddler to overeat. Most young ones will push food away when they are not hungry. By bribing, coaxing, tempting, and teaching our little ones to constantly stuff down a few more bites, they are learning to ignore their body's correct hunger and satiation signals. Over time, and with the help of "fake food" made with artificial flavors and concentrated sweeteners, it's very common for children to become chronic overeaters.

We are designed to consume a diet rich in natural plant fibers and micronutrients. This fiber (bulk) causes stretch receptors in the digestive tract to register that we have consumed enough food. When we eat processed food, which is high in calories and has little fiber, the body's natural satiation mechanism is fooled and we overeat.

Appetite can also be driven by taste. The artificially high stimulation of taste with concentrated sweeteners and artificial flavors can make humans eating machines without constraints.

Man-made, high-calorie concoctions, designed to appeal to the taste and mindset of children, are chemical inventions created to attract consumption, and do not contain the nutrients needed for good health. Besides containing insignificant amounts of nutrients, they also contain potentially dangerous ingredients such as artificial food colorings and chemical preservatives. In addition, processed foods may also contain trans fats, high-fructose corn syrup, sugar, other concentrated sweeteners, white flour, butter, and nitrates. Heavily baked, smoked, or barbequed foods produce heat-formed by-products with detrimental carcinogenic effects. Parents have allowed the processed food and fast food industry to penetrate the minds and bodies of our children like a cult, stealing away the health potential of our children.

THE FIVE MOST DANGEROUS THINGS
TO FEED YOUR CHILD

Butter and cheese—full of saturated fat and fat-delivered chemical pollutants

Potato chips and french fries—rich in trans fat, salt, and carcinogenic acrylamides

Doughnuts and other trans fat–containing sweets—rich in trans fat, sugar, and other artificial substances

Sausages, hot dogs, and other luncheon meats—contain N-nitroso compounds that are potent carcinogens

Pickled, smoked, or barbequed meats—places you at risk of both stomach cancer and high blood pressure

DR. FUHRMAN'S FAB FIVE

Berries—Add berries to morning cereals. Make dessert sorbets from frozen berries. My kids love frozen strawberries blended with an orange or orange juice. We usually add a slice of dried pineapple and use our Vita-Mix to make a smooth and delicious strawberry sorbet.

Greens—Make steamed greens with a cashew butter cream sauce. Kids love it. We blend raw cashews and a few dried onion flakes with some soy milk and make a great sauce for chopped kale or broccoli.

Seeds—Seeds are supernutritious wonder foods. Try sprinkling some lightly toasted unhulled sesame seeds and sunflower seeds on salads and vegetables. We like to grind some into a powder and use it like salt on food.

Beans—Beans are fiber- and nutrient-packed. They give soups that chewy goodness and long-lasting satiety. Add a mixture of split peas, lentils, and adzuki beans to soups and simmer over low heat for about three hours.

Tomatoes—Tomatoes are a wonder food in their own class. Whether you consider them a fruit or a vegetable, it matters not. Slice them into pita pocket sandwiches. Mash some almond butter with a fork into some tomato sauce to add to the vegetable-tomato-sprout-avocado pita pocket. What a great school lunch.

ANIMALS EAT FOR NUTRIENTS

All primates, including humans, are driven to consume food from a variety of categories. Contrary to popular belief, a monkey does not sit under a banana tree eating bananas all day. He eats a few bananas and then may travel half a mile away to find a different type of food. He has an innate drive to consume variety; just satisfying the caloric drive is not enough. Likewise, children will not be satisfied with eating only one or two foods; they will want to eat a portion of one food and want another type of food. As a higher-order animal with a bigger brain, we search for a variety of nutrient sources, and this variety assures that we get the broad assortment of nutrients that increases our immune function and longevity potential. I call this desire for different foods our **variety driver.**

The genetic makeup of humans is not equipped to deal with fake foods. Artificial foods, as well as cheese, oil, fruit juices, and other sweeteners, have cultivated eating habits richer in calories than a primitive diet of natural foods would contain, and one grossly void of immune-system-supporting nutrients. With such unnatural sources of concentrated calories around, we can pack a huge caloric load into a little one's stomach, suppressing their appetite for hours and reducing or eliminating their desire to eat real food. In addition, their innate *variety driver* has been meddled with and no longer directs them to choose appropriate foods.

For instance, some parents think that their children are not eating enough, so they try to entice them with some kind of unwholesome "treat." The minute children taste these low-nutrient processed foods—which are typically high in fat, salt, and sugar—their desire and their taste for wholesome foods diminishes. To the extent that the parents gave in to the attraction of rich, calorically dense foods such as macaroni and cheese, sweets, or pizza, by that same extent, the child will no longer have an interest in consuming fruits and vegetables.

The sense of taste is a very important factor triggering the release of digestive juices and initiating the process of proper digestion. Taste can also be a guide for the body to judge the correct amount of food to consume, providing one is eating natural food. To satisfy true hunger, natural food tastes great. As the appetite is satiated, the thrill of eating diminishes and we feel we have had enough. Yet when we are exposed to processed foods, the body's natural signals to stop eating are disturbed. We offer tasty treats and desserts to stimulate an already-full appetite further and entice all to eat more. Then the unhealthier the diet becomes, the more food addiction plays a role in governing appetite. We feel the need to imbibe when we get accustomed to consuming unhealthful foods. Unhealthful foods are addicting; healthy foods are not, and do not induce overeating.

It is exceedingly rare for a child to eat too little. Yet we are constantly worried that they are not getting enough or that they are too thin. Ninety-nine percent of the time children are coerced by parents to overeat. Never before in world history have so many concoctions been created: pastries, cookies, breads, candies, fried foods, breaded foods, melted cheeses, and other *obesity drivers*.

WHAT IF MY CHILD IS TOO THIN?

We live in a nation of overfed and overweight people, in spite of an overwhelming amount of information that thin people are healthier and live longer. Most doctors are overweight and have overweight children, just like the rest of Americans. They often offer advice that illustrates their ignorance about proper nutrition. Being thin compared to his or her peers does not necessarily mean that your child is not the perfect weight for him or her.

Doctors are trained to detect and investigate the possibility of illness. Certainly, a sudden loss of weight or a sharp decline in expected gains should be looked into to investigate the possibility that there is a developing problem that should be addressed. However, we should also recognize that these problems are exceptionally rare, and in most cases the "too thin" child is at the perfect weight for his or her lean and wiry genetic frame.

I see lots of children whose parents are concerned that they are too thin. In these cases I perform a dietary analysis, confirm that a wholesome well-rounded diet is being followed, and carefully weigh and measure the child. I then assure the parents that their son is not too thin, he is growing normally, and that this body type is his correct genetic structure, which will fill out with more muscular development as he matures.

I have seen many of these healthy "too thin" children develop into beautiful and well-muscled young adults. It just took some time for their muscle-building hormones to kick in. Sometimes they need to do a little weightlifting. Remember that healthy children come in many shapes and sizes.

It is important to be sure that the thin child is not eating sweets and junk food, in other words, the same advice given to an over-weight child. All children have the best opportunity to reach their ideal weight if fed a variety of wholesome natural foods. It is never wise to fill up with poor-quality, disease-causing food in an effort to gain weight.

I have worked as a nutritional advisor to professional and world-class athletes whose nutritional goals are to build muscle mass and fuel athletic strength and stamina. I utilize the same principles to feed normal children. We use an assortment of healthful, natural foods to assure optimal intake of micronutrients, not just calories.

For example, my oldest daughter, Talia, is sixteen years old and a tournament tennis player who trains hard on the tennis court for a few hours each day and then, a few times a week, also works out in the gym. She consumes over 3,000 calories a day and desires to gain muscle and grow more. A sample of her daily menu is a good example of a well-balanced diet for an athlete or somebody de-sirous of weight gain in a healthy manner.

A TYPICAL DAY'S FOOD INTAKE FOR TALIA

....

BREAKFAST
3 cups oatmeal with a chopped apple, ¼ cup raisins, cinnamon,
and 1 tablespoon ground flax seeds.
1 cup unsweetened soy milk
1 persimmon
1 ounce raw sunflower seeds.

LUNCH
Red Hot Hummus* sandwich (2 slices Alvarado Street California
Style Protein Bread with lettuce and tomatoes)
3 cups *Vegetable Pea/Bean Soup**
1 serving *Carob-Avocado Cream Pie**

SNACK
2 frozen bananas blended with ¼ cup soy milk and
1 tablespoon flax seeds
1 oz raw pistachio nuts

DINNER
Large green salad with 6 cups chopped lettuce, 2 tomatoes,
½ cucumber, a slice of red onion, ½ cup raw broccoli,
½ cup snow peas with 2 tablespoons of dressing made from flax
oil, olive oil, balsamic vinegar, and apricot (all fruit) jam
4 cups *California Creamed Kale**
2 Cups *Purple Potato Salad**

*See the recipe section in chapter 5.

ANALYSIS OF THE ABOVE MENU

Nutrient	Actual	Percent RDA
Calories (kcal)	3452	147%
Protein (g)	123	143%
Carbohydrates (g)	548	173%
Fat (g)	113	147%
Saturated fat (g)	17	68%
Cholesterol	79	34%
Total dietary fiber (g)	114	493%
Beta-carotene (IU)	88,227	1765%
Thiamine (mg)	4.8	317%
Riboflavin (mg)	2.9	159%
Niacin (mg)	28	138%
Vitamin B6	7.2	361%
Folate (mcg)	1519	760%
Vitamin C (mg)	610	1017%
Vitamin E (IU)	47	314%
Calcium (mg)	1283	107%
Iron (mg)	40	329%
Magnesium (mg)	1162	290%
Phosphorus (mg)	3112	259%
Selenium (mcg)	140	281%
Sodium (mg)	681	29.5%
Zinc (mg)	20.4	136%

Protein/Carbohydrate/Fat Ratio: 13-59-27

Notes: Vitamin D and B12 requirements are not met by this nearly vegan diet. The much lower than standard recommended amounts of sodium, cholesterol, and saturated fat are of course advantageous. Talia also takes two of my Gentle Care Multivitamins, which give her the extra vitamin D and B12, and one capsule of DHA Purity, a source of vegetable-derived DHA.

By increasing the portion sizes and eating a mixture of vegetables, beans, avocado, nuts, seeds, and fruits, even an athlete in rigorous training can get all the protein and calories she needs. Because there are no "empty calories," the high levels of phytochemical and antioxidants fuel high immune function, so necessary for athletes to avoid illnesses that could derail a promising career.

Those wanting to gain muscle, not fat, should eat similarly. You increase your appetite with exercise and then supply wholesome foods in response to the increased hunger. There is no need to consume extra protein with special powders or shakes; the nutrient-dense food automatically gives you the optimal amount.

REAL FOOD IS AN IMPORTANT PART OF A BALANCED DIET

Once you allow your child to consume the typical American foods, he will reject most, if not all, fresh produce and eat those empty-calorie foods almost exclusively. Your toddler will not have the intellectual maturity to consume broccoli and peas instead of french fries and pizza for his health. The more subtle flavors of natural food can't compete. The pizza, pasta, cheese, burger, and soft drink diet will win over the fruit-vegetable-nut diet seven days of the week.

Furthermore, the unnaturally high level of sugar, salt, and artificially heightened flavors in processed (fake) foods will lessen or deaden the sensitivity of the taste buds to more subtle flavors, making natural foods taste flat. For example, the higher the salt content of your diet, the more your taste buds lose their ability to taste salt. After your taste has toned down its sensitivity to salt, salty things don't taste so salty and your deadened taste buds have lost the ability to enjoy the subtle flavorings in more delicately flavored natural foods. Vegetables have less flavor, fruit isn't as sweet, and nuts taste like wood after just one month of overstimulation with industrial-designed flavors.

Children eat little real food today. By real food, I mean things that are eaten in their natural state. Is an ice pop real food? Are Kool-Aid or macaroni and cheese? Were these foods eaten by primitive man or other primates? Do they contain a reasonable complement of the trace elements, phytochemicals, minerals, and fibers that nature placed in real food? With so much fake food around, why would we expect our children to choose to eat vegetables, fruits, beans, and nuts, those foods that contain all the health-giving nutrients?

If you are committed to your child eating healthfully, there is only one way to do it—make your home off-limits to processed food and low-nutrient foods. No white flour products, no cheese, no sweeteners, no ready-to-eat cereal, no fruit juice, no chips, no junk.

PREPARING YOUR HOME FOR EATING HEALTHFULLY

- Stock your home with a variety of produce, especially fresh fruits, raw vegetables, raw nuts, and seeds. Incorporate bean burgers, vegetable/bean soups, and fruit-centered desserts.

- Replace foods of animal origin with foods of plant origin. Limit poultry to once or twice a week and red meat to even less. Remove skin from poultry. Use the light meat only.

- Remove sugar, salt, and white flour from the home, as well as all products with these added. Use only whole-grain breads and pasta. Use tomato sauce for pasta, not oil-based or cheese-based sauces. Try bean or lentil pasta instead of wheat flour pasta.

- Minimize the use of vegetable oils, replacing them with dressings and sauces made with avocados and whole nuts and seeds. Make delicious desserts with nuts, seeds, and avocados to encourage the consumption of healthy fats.

- Do not keep cheese and butter in the house. If eating dairy foods, select no-fat varieties and only eat small amounts. Replace dairy products with soy milk and nut milk fortified with calcium and vitamin D and B12. If utilizing dairy products in your home, only use fat-free versions.

- Avoid eating lobster, shrimp, mollusks, catfish, swordfish, bluefish, mackerel, pike, shark, tuna, and any fish caught in questionable waters. Limit other fish to once weekly.

- Eliminate fried foods and barbecued foods, both of which expose you to high levels of carcinogenic compounds produced by these high-heat cooking methods.

- Remove all sweet drinks, soda, and processed fruit juice from the house.

- Make healthy snacks available; cherry tomatoes, raw nuts, carrots, fruit, chickpeas, corn, and raw string beans are great choices. (For toddlers below the age of two and a half, be aware of the choking hazard of whole nuts and carrots.)

Don't be concerned if your child doesn't eat much at first, which can be difficult for parents. Rest assured, when your child actually gets hungry he will start eating the assortment of natural foods you

Dr. Fuhrman's Simple Family Food Pyramid

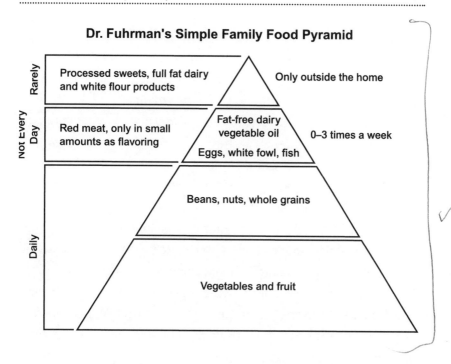

have set out. Eventually your child will consume the same overall number of calories from natural foods that he was previously getting from junk foods. This approach will work even with very picky eaters, because even a relatively sparse assortment of natural foods will provide them with more nutrients than they were getting from their prior diet. Then, in a very short time, both their hunger and their *variety driver* will kick in to lead them to larger portions of phytochemical-rich food and eventually a wider variety of healthy foods.

If you are committed to raising a healthy family without medical tragedies in their future, you must structure your lives so you do not eat in fast food restaurants. Eating outside the home should be a rare occurrence. Parents should pack their kids' school lunches and plan family meals together as much as possible. Dinner together should be a time for all to model healthy eating and counter the influence of the fake food culture with good nutrition.

In a home environment bursting with real food, food no longer needs to become an issue. Let your children eat as much or as little as they want. A normal child will self-regulate and consume a healthy diet, given a healthy home environment.

There is solid evidence to establish the ability of children to control their caloric intake and food selection. However, this does not mean that children can do this in today's toxic food environment. Children can't be expected to devise a wholesome balanced diet when faced with so many unnatural and unhealthy choices. Nevertheless, research on this point demonstrates that when children are left alone to adjust their own caloric intake without parental control, the children maintain a very consistent level of caloric intake even in the face of changing the types of food and caloric density of the food offered.[8] This means that the best way to prevent overeating or undereating is to let the child be in charge of how much or how little he eats.

THE FORBIDDEN FRUIT SYNDROME

Another reason we should not continually battle with our children about how much and what we want them to eat is that it does not work effectively. Teaching them about the value and consequences of eating healthy food is important, but it should not be taught by forcing something down their throat.

If you set an example of healthful eating practices and all in the house participate in discussing the reasons why you live that way, the rules will be respected and not seem arbitrary. If you try to force your child to eat one way while you eat another way, he will be too young to understand why he is doing it, but eating will become a battle. If there is unhealthy food in the house it will become the "forbidden fruit," and the attraction of eating what they shouldn't is magnified.

We shouldn't try to control what children eat; rather, we need to direct their food intake. Kids generally learn to eat the foods their parents do. We control their food options by what we have in the home. Kids will choose well when they are in the right environment. As parents we must create the right environment and limit their exposure to the wrong environment.

We wouldn't want our children living in a cocaine-snorting or pot-smoking household, would we? We would not take children to parties with heavy drinking and drug use. Shooting up with drugs, getting drunk, and even smoking are unhealthy behaviors, and children will mimic their parents' behaviors regardless of the warnings given. Unfortunately, it is socially dictated to get together with friends and recreate with alcohol, soda, and junk food and stuff yourself to the point of discomfort. If you do this on a regular basis, you will teach that to your children, too. Cultivate friends who value their health and who support your chosen lifestyle.

Control your children's environment, limit their exposure to junk food, teach them about nutrition, and then as they get older allow them to make their own choices in the real world, outside the home. You may be surprised at how wise they are. As they have become older, my children are in more and more situations where poor food choices are present, and they choose to limit their consumption of unhealthy food. They are extremely sensible, but not perfect. It makes common sense to them to take proper care of their bodies, as they learned that eating right was a gift that parents give their children when they are loved, to protect their future. The ongoing sharing of information about life, ethics, art, education, and nutrition can be interwoven into the education they receive in the home in an entertaining, caring, and loving manner.

An important point to emphasize is that you should not purchase and bring into the home foods that you do not want your children to be eating. For example, if you buy ice cream and eat it, it makes no sense and is counterproductive to restrict your children from eating it. One sensible alternative is to have ice cream only outside the home, at a party or special occasion when the whole family has it together. Children understand that the reason it is consumed rarely is because it is not a safe food to consume more frequently. When eaten on a special occasion together there is no guilt or hidden "cheating" involved. In place of ice cream in the home, healthy desserts and ice cream made predominantly with fresh and frozen fruits can be eaten and enjoyed as much as high-fat, artificially sweetened, or sugary ice cream.

THE SECRETS TO GETTING YOUR CHILDREN TO EAT HEALTHFULLY

1. Keep only healthy food in the house. Every person in the household should have the same food choices available.

2. Offer and feed a wholesome diversity of natural foods, vegetables, beans, raw nuts, seeds, and fresh fruits, while giving each child as much latitude as possible to eat what they prefer.

3. Don't attempt to manage your children's caloric intake. They can do that on their own.

4. If you, as parents, do not demonstrate proper respect for your own bodies by eating healthy, exercising regularly, and engaging in other healthful lifestyle practices, don't expect your children to do any better than you, now or in the future.

5. Educate your children about their nutritional needs and the importance of eating healthfully. Start this when they are young and continue to reinforce their learning, as they will

be exposed to more toxic food choices as they get older
and spend more time out of their home.

It is important to realize that it is never too late to teach your children the importance of eating healthy. As you learn, share it enthusiastically with them. Work on improving your diets together. If
your child is a teenager, let her read what you are reading. You may
want to add that it will help their complexion and body shape. Even
teenagers will make beneficial improvements in their diets when
presented with compelling reasons. I have lectured to high school
assemblies many times and am always impressed by how interested, enthusiastic, and willing to make changes teenagers can be.
Research supports this willingness of adolescents to make significant dietary change when presented with accurate and compelling
information.[9]

One study educating girls about food and health showed that the
girls' hormone levels during puberty were cut by about 50 percent
when taught about eating healthier.[10] Dr. Stevens, a psychologist
involved with the study, made the following conclusion:

> The key to getting your kids to eat healthfully is to control
> what food is in the house and to show by example, said psy-
> chologist Stevens. He continued, "Even with teenagers, con-
> trolling the food that is in the house is the top strategy for
> getting kids to eat more healthfully. If you have junk food in
> the house, they will eat it. If there is fruit, they will eat that.
> But if you show them you are eating healthy, they will most
> likely eat that way too."

The first step toward your child's healthy eating is changing your
own. Concentrate on changing the dietary habits of the parents first
and gradually remove more and more of the unhealthy options. If

your child doesn't change his diet the first day, that is okay. Stop trying to control his intake. Stop battling. Instead, continue to offer delicious vegetable dishes and other great foods that are available. If he chooses to eat very little of it, that is fine. The best way to handle it is to say, "You don't have to eat. If you are not hungry, why don't you go and play." If he asks for something not in the house, simply tell him that you do not have any. When he gets very hungry, he will ask to eat and relish what was offered earlier. You might be surprised at how much good stuff he will eat because he is really hungry and not forced to eat something when he was not. It will also be easier if he sees the rest of the family enjoying eating the healthy food choices and healthful recipes.

YOUR CHILD ALREADY KNOWS
HOW MUCH TO EAT

The vast majority of children eat the precise amount of calories they need for excellent health. Given the availability of real food that contains nutrients, their bodies will give them normal signals that will control the amount and even diversity of food for them to maintain excellent health. Left to their own devices, toddlers eat when they are hungry and consume more food during growth spurts and times of heavy activity. In other words, they adjust their caloric intake to match their needs. They typically do a better job at it than adults do. And they certainly do a better job at it than parents who try to decide for their kids how much the child needs to eat.

Their hunger can't be denied, so your child cannot eat too little. The stomach fills up quickly on healthy choices, so your child cannot eat too much. A natural food diet style ends both under-eating and overeating. It promotes a normal relationship with food that will continue later in life and will offer long-lasting disease protection.

Hunger is the cue to eat, but in our society, the clock has become our cue. We expect our children to be hungry at the exact moment we have the meal ready and not before or later. *"Don't eat before dinner; it will spoil your appetite,"* is a common admonition. That is like saying, Even if you are hungry now, I want you to suffer until dinner is served. A snack an hour before dinner does not have to be forbidden as long as they are making healthy choices. However, since I don't want to discourage the concept of a family meal, consider this: if they are hungry and request food before dinner, offer your children the lower-calorie snacks, such as fruit and raw vegetables, so they still have an appetite left for dinner.

If children are not hungry at dinner, they should not be pressured to eat more. When we say, "You have to clean your plate or you can't go outside and play" we mean, "Force that food down, even if you are not hungry." The groundwork for a lifetime battle with food is being put into place.

We teach our children to eat when not hungry. We encourage it. Many parents actually think it looks healthy for their kids to be plump and bigger than average. They continually encourage them to ignore their bodies and eat when not hungry. The children learn to eat for a taste thrill; it is recreational eating, akin to recreational drug use. They do it for a thrill and pay a price for it later. These children and adults have overeaten their whole lives, so that they have no recollection of what true hunger feels like.

THE CONCEPT OF "TOXIC HUNGER"

Losing your ability to sense true hunger sets the foundation for obesity. By feeding them so much calorie-rich food so frequently we have trained our children to disconnect eating from hunger. After enough time goes by continually consuming more calories than they need, they will feel discomfort when they do not have food constantly in their stomach. They must keep their digestive tract going all the time, because the minute it empties, they feel uncomfortable. By the time they become an overweight adult, they are true food addicts.

A few hours after eating, feeling weak, headachy, tired, mentally dull, and stomach cramping or discomfort is not true hunger! These symptoms of stomach cramping and fluttering, headaches and fatigue that begin when digestion is completed I call "toxic hunger" because these symptoms only occur in those who have been eating a toxic diet. These are withdrawal symptoms from an unhealthful diet, and this discomfort is mistakenly interpreted as the need to eat more frequently and take in more calories. Continual eating stops the discomfort, just like frequent coffee drinking stops the headaches from caffeine withdrawal. Your body can't withdraw from (detoxify and repair) your toxic dietary habits and digest a meal simultaneously. By eating, this detox process is stopped. When we consume a toxic, disease-promoting diet, our body reacts in an attempt to remove or deal with the damage this unhealthful diet could cause. This concept is called withdrawal. The body attempts to detoxify from a harmful, low-nutrient diet and we feel the symptoms of toxic hunger. We build up more waste products in our cells when we eat unhealthfully, and when the body is not busy digesting, it can attempt to withdraw from or initiate repair mechanisms that result in these uncomfortable symptoms. The disease-building diet most Americans eat drives these symptoms, and these symptoms promote overeating.

Symptoms of Toxic Hunger

- headaches

- fatigue

- nausea

- weakness

- mental confusion

- abdominal and esophageal spasm

- fluttering and cramping

True hunger is felt in the neck and throat; where thirst is felt, hunger is a subtle sensation, and when you feel it, almost any food tastes good and satisfies you. True hunger is not felt in the head or belly. When you eat when you are truly hungry, your ability to taste is maximized and food truly tastes better. True hunger marks the time when the digestive juices are ready to be released and the enzyme-secreting glands have had time to refill and are ready for action. Healthy digestion, not indigestion, results. When we eat only when hungry, we also prevent ourselves from becoming over-weight and maximize our chances for a long, disease-free life.

Our body has the beautifully orchestrated ability to give us the precise signals to tell us exactly how much to eat to maintain an ideal weight for our long-term health. In an environment of healthy food choices, we would not feel any hunger until the hormonal and neurological messengers indicated that the glycogen reserves in the liver were decreasing.

Satisfying our body's signals of true hunger dictates that we eat sufficiently to maintain our lean body mass and no more. One cannot become overweight satisfying true hunger. To gain fat on your body, you have to eat more than hunger demands. When food addictions drive intake via toxic hunger, we are never satisfied with an empty stomach, because it feels too uncomfortable, so we eat more and more and invariably become overweight. The more unhealthy the diet is, the more toxic hunger drives the person to overeat and put on additional pounds. It is a vicious cycle. In childhood, children get trained to overeat, and by the time they reach adulthood they are addicted to overeating and get heavier and heavier.

Dieting, or trying to eat less food, is not an effective way for adults to lose weight, either. The best diet isn't one at all. If you eat large amounts of healthful, nutrient-rich foods, you will lose the toxic hunger sensations and get back in touch with true hunger signals. Then you will be able to stop the food cravings and munchies for the first time in your life. Not eating when not hungry is a crucial starting point for successful weight control. When you eat enough healthy food and stop the junk food, the body naturally regulates its hunger response to maintain your ideal weight.

INSTILLING GOOD EATING HABITS IN YOUR CHILD

It is fine to abandon the "three meals a day" tradition; it is okay to let children eat twice or six times a day. Let your children have a say in what and when they will eat. Abandon the myths, the traditions, and the difficulty in attempting to control your child's biological drives.

Parents are entrusted with the responsibility of securing the selection of healthy foods for the family and preparing the food in a way that makes it desirable. Children are responsible for deciding how much they eat. If they are in an environment of healthful foods they will have no problem regulating variety and timing. They can choose what they eat, when they eat, and if they will eat.

Don't use food as a reward or punishment. Don't offer a treat because the child was good or ate well. Offer healthy treats as part of the normal well-balanced diet.

If the family is having an "outside," more conventional treat on occasion, don't teach your child that it is because of an achievement. If children are rewarded and comforted with cookies and ice cream, it builds emotional attachment to these foods. Special foods

FIVE HEALTHY TREATS

1. **Date nut pop-ems**—A mix of dates, ground nuts, cinnamon, and carob powder

2. **Soaked dried fruit**—Dried apricots, apples, or mangoes soaked overnight in soy milk

3. **Frozen banana whip**—Frozen bananas, sliced and pureed in a blender or food processor with a little soy milk or skim milk

4. **Baked apples**—Cored apples filled with a mix of apple sauce, cinnamon, and raisins and then baked at 350 degrees for 20 minutes

5. **Fruit smoothies**—A blended mixture of fresh fruit, banana, dried fruit, and soy milk, milk, or fruit juice. Unsweetened canned pineapple, with the juice mixed with banana and frozen strawberries, is a kid favorite. Experiment.

should be for holidays and the outside-the-home special occasion, not as a prize.

If childhood memories of vegetables include being forced to choke down peas, it does not help to nurture positive feelings and an affinity toward the taste of peas. Children will learn to enjoy these foods best by watching adults appreciate the flavors and health benefits in a subtle manner, which will lead to a lifetime appreciation of vegetables prepared in a variety of interesting ways.

Here is the most important rule: ***No rules only for children.*** If the parents are not willing to follow the rules set for the house, they should not be imposed on the children. Don't argue about what your children should and shouldn't be eating; discuss this in private. As parents, we must be consistent, but not perfect. Likewise, it is okay for the children to be consistent, but not perfect either. For example, if the parents decide that an unhealthy food or a restaurant meal is acceptable for the children once per week, then that goes for the adults, too. Setting an example supported by both parents is the most important and most effective way for your children to develop a healthy attitude toward food.

Parents must decide on the standards they want to set in their home. They should educate themselves, then come to an agreement about which foods are permitted and which are not. Whenever possible, consider your children's input. Menus, school lunches, and planning what foods to purchase at the market should all be decided in advance to accommodate the likes and food preferences of all in the family. When you work together for the same goal as a family unit, you can encourage and help each other to eat healthier. Children can help parents, too.

Barbara Fox had been seeing me as a patient for two years. She liked receiving my nutritional guidance to manage her diabetes because before she came to me her sugars were climbing and her prior doctor wanted to start her on insulin. We were able to control her blood sugar, and I encouraged her to exercise and make more significant changes in her diet. I shared with Barbara stories of the hundreds of patients who have completely reversed diabetes and are no longer diabetic because of my nutritional advice. She was intrigued, but did not change her eating habits enough to lose substantial weight; she was still diabetic. What changed Barbara and enabled her to lose sixty-five pounds and rid herself of her diabetes was her sixteen-year-old daughter, Caroline. Barbara brought Caroline to see me for chronic migraine headaches. Caroline had seen several headache specialists and had been prescribed more and more drugs, but they were working less and less. She did not want to be on so much medication, and after Barbara spoke to another patient who had vanquished headaches with my advice, Caroline came to see me. I slowly weaned Caroline off of all her headache medications and started her on a high-nutrient, natural food diet. Her headaches slowly resolved and disappeared for good. At the same time, Barbara began to eat the super healthy diet I had prescribed for Caroline. They were a support system for each other, and over the next fifteen months Barbara lost sixty-five pounds. She no longer required any medications for diabetes.

Again and again, I have seen children help their parents lose weight and get well from diseases such as diabetes, high blood pressure, and allergies. Children eating healthfully was usually the death blow to the parents' unhealthy eating. Given the right information, children are often very smart about eating right. When they do, they often encourage the parents to take better care of themselves, too.

PARENTING YOUR CHILD IN THE KITCHEN

The entire family should help with food preparation if possible, which can also be a good time to discuss food issues and educate the children about eating healthfully. Involve your young children in food preparation by giving them something to do. Let them mash a banana or stir a bowl of food. When they are involved, they will be more connected to eating the food they helped prepare. Your toddler will want to eat the foods you made together and those you eat together. Share these dishes proudly made by the children with the rest of the family.

Because a child's diet during the first ten years of life is so important, it should be reassuring to see how young children easily learn to love healthy food. Fruits and vegetables are the foods they are naturally most attracted to—if given the chance.

Remember, you and your children are not following a diet. As a family, you have chosen a new way of eating to improve your health and enjoyment of food. You can all work together to have healthy food available and to make it taste great. This lifestyle is chosen because of wisdom, the exposure to new scientific information, and the love you all have for each other. No matter what age your children are now, they will respect you and appreciate your loving concern. They will likely pass this knowledge and practice on to their own children.

There is no special discipline required; eating good-tasting food that just happens to be good for you, too, is not hard; it is pleasurable. It does take some effort to learn the information, modify the recipes you usually make, and work together as a family to eat better.

Early exposure to an assortment of fresh fruits, vegetables, and raw nuts is an important component of your child's future health. If you make squash for the family and your toddler turns his head away from it, don't give up. Serve squash again that week. Let your child see the rest of the family eating it, and then make a fuss over how good it is and offer some to your child again. If he refuses to taste it, or tastes it and spits it out, do not give up; continue to repeat the above scenario over and over.

Remember, it takes eight to fifteen tastes for a child to develop a liking for a new food. Keep trying to have your child taste the healthy foods the rest of the family is eating. Most parents find that they have no problem getting their young children to eat plenty of vegetables.

As your child gets older, birthday cake and other unhealthy foods might be offered on occasion. If no fuss is made and nothing discussed, three things might occur: the child might have a few bites and nothing more, she might eat the whole piece, or she might not even like the sweet or artificial taste.

My daughter Cara found birthday cake distasteful. We always

fed our children a good meal of their favorite foods before they left the house prior to birthday parties or other events to make sure they were not hungry when exposed to this kind of food. By the time they were older and faced with parents distributing soda and doughnuts at soccer games, they were already knowledgeable enough to say no thank you on their own. They knew the health consequences of such eating habits.

If your children choose to eat junk on occasion, let it go. Try not to make them feel bad about it. You will know how healthfully they eat when they are home, which should be more than 90 percent of their intake. Control what is done in the home, and make sure that 90 percent of the time the family is eating at home. The best approach is to control what you can control and don't try to control what you can't.

The goal is for your children to eat healthfully because they want to, and do so whether their parents are around or not. We need to respect their decisions as they mature and give them the leeway to formulate their decision to eat healthfully because they want to. The reasons to do so are compelling. By educating them and being good examples, they will simply follow suit. In the same way, your children should learn to enjoy exercise. If parents exercise and engage in sports for fun and recreation, so will their children.

It is not harmful to a child's self-esteem, nor will it lead to unfounded fears, anxiety, or eating disorders, to learn about the harmful effects of disease-causing foods. Right now, it is socially acceptable to teach children about the dangers of drugs and smoking. But it has not yet become politically correct to educate our children about the potential dangers of the typical disease-causing diets and disease-causing foods. Never before in human history have we had such a huge availability and exposure to "fake foods" and rich foods that make eating poorly so common that we guarantee more and more adults suffering from autoimmune system disorders such as lupus, colitis, arthritis, and even multiple sclerosis. It is time to elevate the consciousness of people to put an end to this socially promoted destruction of the next generation.

IS IT HEALTHIER FOR MY CHILDREN TO BE ON A VEGETARIAN OR VEGAN DIET, OR A MIXED OMNIVOROUS DIET?

All types of diets—vegetarian or non-vegetarian—have potential health risks as well as associated benefits. My patients frequently ask me questions about the positive aspects and the dangers of different types of diets. Here's how eating styles are defined:

- **Vegan**—one whose diet is totally from plant foods, with no dairy, eggs, or other foods of animal origin.

- **Vegetarian**—one whose diet avoids eating animals, but may or may not include some dairy, eggs, or other.

- **Omnivorous**—eating both animal products and plant foods.

- **Lacto-ovo vegetarian**—one whose diet contains no meat, fowl, or fish, but who uses eggs and dairy products.

When looking for the healthiest diet to promote a long life free of disease, we must first consider a vegetarian or vegan diet. There are two things we all know with certainty. First of all, a diet rich in vegetables, beans, fruits, raw nuts, and seeds has a dramatic effect on reducing the risk of both heart disease and most cancers. The other thing we know is that as animal products increase in a population's diet, the risk of developing heart disease and cancer increases. It has been observed in multiple scientific studies that vegetarians have

fewer heart attacks and less incidence of cancer than those on omnivorous diets.

The chief feature that makes a vegetarian diet beneficial compared to more conventional ways of eating is that a person following a vegetarian diet is more likely to consume more high-nutrient
produce that contains protective fibers and antioxidant nutrients,
and the diet will naturally be lower in saturated fat, which is a
known risk factor for both heart disease and cancer.

Not surprisingly, fruits and vegetables are the two foods with the
highest correlation with longevity in humans. Not whole wheat
bread, not bran, not even a vegetarian diet shows as powerful a correlation with decreased mortality as does a high level of fresh fruit
and raw green vegetable consumption.[11] The National Cancer Institute recently reported on 337 different studies, with all showing the
same basic information:[12]

1. Vegetables and fruits protect against all types of cancers if
   consumed in large enough quantities. Thousands of scientific
   studies document this. The most prevalent cancers in our
   country are primarily plant-food deficiency diseases.

2. Raw vegetables have the most powerful anti-cancer
   properties of all foods.

3. Beans, in general, and not just soy, have additional
   anti-cancer benefits against reproductive cancers like breast
   and prostate cancer.

Clearly the chief health reason to choose a vegetarian diet is to
consume high levels of fruits, green vegetables, and beans. This is the
key to both better health and healthy weight loss. This still begets the
question that is often asked: Is it absolutely necessary to follow a
vegetarian diet to achieve protection from common diseases and

achieve excellent health? The answer is no, a very small amount of animal products can be utilized and a small amount of oil can be utilized without placing oneself at risk, but these foods should be significantly limited.

A vegetarian whose diet is mainly refined grains, cold breakfast cereals, processed health food store products, vegetarian fast foods, white rice, and pasta will be worse off than a person who eats a little turkey, chicken, fish, or eggs but consumes large volumes of fruits, vegetables, and beans. That combination of little or no animal products with a higher consumption of fresh produce is the crucial factor that makes a vegetarian diet healthful. There are plenty of vegans who eat diets rich in oils, salt, and processed vegan food, and are still overweight or in poor health. Simply being a vegetarian does not make one healthier unless that person is actually eating healthy foods. There are lots of unhealthy vegetarian foods and unhealthy vegetarians.

Even though most studies have shown that vegetarians live longer than non-vegetarians do, it does not mean that all vegetarians do so well.[13] We know the research shows that those who avoid meat and dairy have lower rates of heart disease, cancer, high blood pressure, diabetes, and obesity, which are the leading causes of death in America.[14] But when we take a close look at the data, it appears that those who weren't as strict at avoiding animal products entirely had longevity statistics that were equally impressive—as long as they consumed high volumes of a variety of unrefined plant foods. In other words, you can achieve the benefits of a vegetarian diet without being a total vegan, and the science available seems to support this.

Don't miss the important point I am trying to stress here. Whether you eat a vegetarian diet or you include a very small amount of animal foods, for optimal health you must get the majority of calories from unrefined plant food with a minimal amount of animal products. A large quantity of unrefined plant food grants the greatest protection against developing serious disease.

One may choose to be on a healthy vegetarian diet, with careful planning, and one can choose to be on a healthy omnivorous diet with careful planning, too. Both ways of eating still require knowledge about nutrition, to assure excellent health and disease protection.

DRAWBACKS OF A VEGETARIAN DIET

A strict vegetarian or vegan diet has certain drawbacks that are easily remedied. Vegan food is deficient in meeting the nutrient needs of most individuals for vitamin B12. If you or your children are following a complete vegetarian (vegan) diet, it is essential that you consume a multivitamin or a B12 source such as fortified soymilk.

Vitamin D, often called the sunshine vitamin, is another potential deficiency in those not drinking vitamin D–fortified milk. Synthetic vitamin D is added to both cow's milk and most brands of soy milk today.

Most of us adults work indoors and avoid the sun or wear sunscreens, which lowers our vitamin D exposure. Some of us live in northern climates, are not outdoors as much, don't absorb it as well, or just require more. It is important to assure that your vitamin D requirements are met sufficiently. Infants and toddlers spend most of their time indoors, and it is important that children this young do not damage their delicate skin with sun exposure. It is difficult to put sunscreen on toddlers and not safe to use chemical sunscreen on infants. I recommend nonchemical sunscreens on young children made only with titanium and zinc oxide. Nevertheless, the reduced sun exposure makes meeting vitamin D requirements with food or supplements essential.

It is especially important that young children receive vitamin D because a deficiency of it can cause bone abnormalities. Vitamin D is transmitted via breast milk as long as the mother's stores are adequate. But as breast-feeding diminishes and children receive most of their calories from food, it is important to assure that they get vitamin D in the diet. So if breast-feeding, the mother's vitamin D status is important, and if not breast-feeding, there should be an alternative vitamin D source such as formula or vitamin D–fortified soy milk or a children's multivitamin with adequate vitamin D.

It is a myth that a vegetarian diet, rich in green vegetables, beans, and whole grains, would likely be low in calcium or protein. Plant foods contain adequate levels of these nutrients. However, if a vegetarian diet is not carefully designed to include foods such as nuts, seeds, green vegetables, beans, and whole grains, then levels of calcium, iron, zinc, and protein could be low.

For example, iron-deficiency anemia has been reported in some macrobiotic vegetarians who followed a very restrictive diet and consumed a diet with rice as their staple food. This iron deficiency would not have occurred if these individuals had eaten more green vegetables and beans, which contain adequate iron.

A natural-food-based vegetarian diet does not cause iron-deficiency anemia, it gives you the ideal amount. By the way, chicken and turkey do not have much iron in them. Vegetables and beans have much more.

COMPARISON OF IRON SOURCES

Food	Iron (mg/100 calories)
Spinach, cooked	5.4
Collard greens, cooked	3.1
Lentils, cooked	2.7
Broccoli, cooked	2.1

Chickpeas, cooked	1.7
Raw cashews	1.7
Sirloin steak, choice, broiled	1.6
White potato, baked	1.3
Figs, dried	0.8
Hamburger, lean, broiled	0.8
Chicken, roasted, no skin	0.6
Turkey, breast	0.4
Blueberries	0.4
Flounder, baked	0.3
Pork chop, pan-fried	0.2
Milk, skim	0.1

If vegetarians and vegans eat a variety of plant proteins, their intake of protein should be as good as that of a person who eats meat or other foods that contain animal protein. The mixture of proteins from grains, legumes, seeds, nuts, and vegetables provides a complement of amino acids so that deficits in one food are made up by another.

Not all types of plant foods need to be eaten at the same meal, since the amino acids are combined in the body's protein pool. So there is no need to mix or match amino acids to form a complete protein at each meal; your body can do that on its own from what you consume all day.

Keep in mind that it is not a vegetarian diet per se that is low in these aforementioned nutrients; it is that some who indiscriminately drop animal products from their diet may not substitute enough of the nutrient-rich plant foods to make the diet adequate.

SALT MAY BE EVEN MORE TOXIC TO VEGANS
AND VEGETARIANS

Although a low-saturated-fat vegan diet may markedly reduce risk for coronary heart disease, diabetes, and many common cancers, the real Achilles' heel of the low-fat vegan diet is the increased risk of hemorrhagic (vessel rupture leading to bleeding) stroke at a late age. Apparently the atherosclerotic (plaque-building) process that creates a local vascular environment favorable to coronary thrombosis (clot) and intravascular embolism (traveling clot) may be protecting the fragile blood vessels in the brain from rupture under years of stress from high blood pressure. Admittedly, hemorrhagic stroke causes a very small percentage of deaths in modern countries. It still is worth noting that if strict vegetarians are to have the potential to maximize their lifespan, it is even more important for them to avoid a high salt intake because salt intake increases blood pressure. Almost all of the soy-based meat analogues and many other health food store (vegan) products are exceptionally high in sodium.

A number of studies both in Japan (where the high-salt diet had made stroke a leading cause of death) and in the West have illustrated that fewer animal products and a low serum cholesterol were associated with an increased risk of hemorrhagic stroke.[15] Keep in mind, stroke mortality is significantly higher in Japan and exceptionally high in certain areas of China where salt intake is high, in spite of low-fat diets. It is also well established that Third World countries that do not salt their food are virtually immune to hypertension, the age-related rise in blood pressure we see in 90 percent of Americans, and they are immune to the incidence of strokes.

The high salt→high blood pressure→stroke causation chain may be more likely a late-life event in a vegetarian successfully maintaining excellent heart health. So avoiding excess sodium may be even more important for a vegetarian than for an omnivore. Of course, excess sodium increases both heart attack and stroke death in all diet styles, but in a vegan, the high-salt diet is even more likely to rear its ugly head as a cause of late-life morbidity and mortality, especially since they will often live longer and not have a heart attack first.

DHA FAT (FISH OIL) MAY BE LOW WHEN NOT EATING FISH

Another concern is that many vegetarians and others who do not eat fish may not have ideal levels of all essential fatty acids. Fish supply two nonessential fatty acids, EPA and DHA, that have been shown to have beneficial effects, offering protection against both heart disease and aging of the brain. They are called "nonessential" fats because the body can make EPA and DHA from the short-chain omega-3 fats found in nuts, seeds, and greens. To ensure that vegetarians get sufficient levels of these omega-3 fats, they need to consume foods such as flax seeds, hemp seeds, and walnuts on a regular basis. Then the body can take these short-chain fatty acids and convert them into the longer-chain (EPA and DHA) fats typically found in fish.

The problem is that people vary in their ability to convert short-chain omega-3 fatty acids into DHA. Therefore, some individuals may not have optimal levels of long-chain omega-3 fats (EPA and DHA) even with the consumption of a well-designed vegetarian diet utilizing omega-3-fat-containing seeds and nuts. There is an overwhelming amount of evidence today that adequate nutrition, including a high level of plant-derived antioxidants as well as adequate DHA, is important to maximize health and to prevent aging of the brain.[16]

Some will argue that the body can produce all the DHA it needs on its own, without supplementation, just from the beneficial fats in nuts and greens. This may be true for a certain percentage of the population, but we all have varying genetic potential to manufacture optimal levels of DHA. To assure that all of us and almost all children get the best possible nutritional building blocks for brain function, I recommend we stack the deck in our favor and take a DHA supplement for solid nutritional insurance.

It is especially helpful for the child's brain development as well as to prevent postpartum depression that pregnant and nursing mothers take a DHA supplement in addition to their multivitamin. This will ensure that the breast milk will contain adequate DHA. Children weaned from the breast should also have a source of DHA in their diet, such as a children's liquid DHA supplement or a multivitamin containing DHA. I would make these same recommendations to everyone, whether they consume a vegetarian or omnivorous diet.

Fish, which is the natural source of DHA, is simply too polluted a food to rely on as a DHA source for children. I do not recommend feeding young children fish in an attempt to supply them with their requirements of DHA. Instead, I recommend taking a clean DHA supplement and avoiding the possibility of mercury and petrochemical pollution found in most fish. Avoiding these pollutants is more important in infants, toddlers, and children, as their growing cells are more sensitive to the damaging effects of toxic pollutants.

Once your child is off breast milk, I recommend that parents add a small amount of DHA (50 to 100 mg) to their child's orange juice, oatmeal, or other food. Even if you do not do it every day, it still ensures that no child will suffer the consequences of DHA deficiency during these crucial years of brain development.

DRAWBACKS OF AN OMNIVOROUS DIET

Much of the people in the modern world today eat a diet that is poorly designed to maximize human health. In fact, the incidence of heart disease, stroke, and cancer is higher in more developed countries and kills the vast majority of all adults, despite the fact that the nutritional causes of these illnesses have been adequately explained by scientific studies.

Nearly the entire populations in developed countries today suffer from diseases of nutritional extravagance leading to an epidemic of obesity, diabetes, and heart disease and a premature death. While Americans jump from one diet craze to another, their waistlines and leading causes of death change little because the popular diets appeal to the most popular way to eat, consuming animal products, oils, and dairy at every meal. The most commercially successful diet books in our country appeal to America's love affair with saturated-fat-rich animal products and still leave the public with a dangerous solution to their growing waistlines. These books encourage a high percentage of animal products in spite of the preponderance of evidence showing the links to heart disease and cancer.

There are three main problems with diets that contain significant amounts of animal products:

1. More than a thousand well-designed studies have led all major health authorities around the world to conclude that saturated fat is a leading contributor to high cholesterol, heart disease, and many cancers.

2. Fat-soluble petrochemicals such as PCBs and dioxin, as well as other toxic elements such as mercury, are transferred to humans predominantly via the fatty portions of fish, dairy, meat, and poultry, and in that order. Fatty fish that are rich sources of omega-3 fats are also typically heavily contaminated with harmful pollutants. These pollutants are linked to neurological problems, immune system dysfunction, and cancer.

3. Animal products contain no fiber, and almost no antioxidant
   vitamins such as vitamins C, K, E, and folate. They also are
   lacking in all the anti-cancer phytochemicals,
   bioflavonoids, lignins, and carotenoids that are so essential
   to protect us against chronic illnesses, immune system
   disorders, and a premature death.

With animal products occupying a major caloric percentage of
the diet, less remains for natural, unrefined plant produce. The inclusion of sugar, white flour, oil, and other low-nutrient calories in
an omnivorous diet virtually guarantees phytonutrient deficiency
and greatly increases the risk of late-life cancer.

The low levels of certain essential nutrients are inevitable unless
an omnivorous diet is designed to receive the vast majority of its
calories from fruits, vegetables, beans, raw nuts, and seeds to supply crucial food elements necessary for optimal health. The amount
of animal products must be held to much lower amounts than are
presently consumed, and those animal products chosen must be
very low in saturated fat and pollutants. The animal products that
are lowest in saturated fat are egg whites, low-fat fish, skinless
white meat turkey, and chicken. The highest saturated-fat animal
products are butter, cheeses, and red meat.

If you choose to include animal products in your diet and your
children's diet, they should be utilized sparingly, as condiments or
flavorings for soups and vegetable dishes, not as the main dish. Use
one piece of chicken to flavor a vegetable bean soup that will be used
for the whole family all week. Use fresh turkey breast sliced very thin
in a sandwich with avocado or tomato-based dressing, lettuce,
tomato, and red onion. In other words, only use one or two ounces a
day per person. A pound of animal product can be used for an entire
family of five for a few days, so that the family's diet is comprised of
vegetables, fruits, beans, and nuts with only a few ounces of animal

products every few days. I call this a near-vegetarian diet. It allows for more variety and flavor in cooking and recipes without losing the main health advantages of a plant-based diet.

Because animal products do not contain significant omega-3 fat, and fatty fish are such a polluted food, it is important for those on an omnivorous diet to consume walnuts, flax, hemp, and other plant sources of omega-3. The valuable omega-3 fats should not be derived from the regular consumption of fatty fish. Instead, I recommend the lower-fat (less polluted) fish such as flounder, sole, and tilapia. Utilizing plant sources of omega-3 such as flax seeds and walnuts is still important. Because the contamination level in fish is always questionable, even these less polluted fish should be used sparingly, just like all other animal products.

A multivitamin and a DHA supplement are still a good idea, for the assurance that optimal levels of these nutrients are met.

VEGETARIAN OR VEGAN DIETS: SAFE FOR CHILDREN?

A diet optimally designed for adult humans would naturally be ideal for the children of that species, too. There are no special needs children have that would make them require a different diet. Even at the time of rapid growth and brain development, the optimal supply of energy and essential fats can be met by an appropriately planned vegetarian or vegan diet. According to the American Dietetic Association and the Institute of Food Technologists, vegan diets can provide adequate nutrition for children.

In May 1998, the seventh edition of *Dr. Spock's Baby and Child Care* was published. In it, Dr. Spock recommends a vegan diet for children. Dr. Spock was concerned that the diet we fed our children, rich in animal products and dairy fat, set them up for adult

diseases and a premature death. He wasn't wrong, but his noncon-
formist view sparked a long-overdue discussion about the scientific
and practical issues of optimal diets for children.

Clearly children of all ages need an adequate supply of healthy
fats to fuel their growth and energy needs and for brain development. Some people believe that even a vitamin B12–supplemented
vegan or vegetarian diet would not supply enough essential fats to
maximize healthy development of the brain. This could be a concern if the diet was all high-carbohydrate foods such as bread, potatoes, rice, and fruit.

The American Academy of Pediatrics recommends that kids
consume 30 percent of their daily calories from fats, with 50 to 55
percent of calories coming from carbohydrates and the remaining
10 to 15 percent from protein. Even if you use these narrow ranges
as a guide, you get that level of fat when you utilize the recipes and
menu plans in this book. Raw nuts, seeds, and avocados are rich in
fat, protein, vitamins, and minerals. Remember, whole nuts such
as peanuts should be avoided in young children, as the shape
makes them possible to get stuck in a toddler's windpipe if not
chewed. But nuts can be safely included in the diet after nine
months of age utilizing nut butters, dressing, sauces, and desserts
to meet these concerns of fat adequacy. Of course, with the growing incidence of peanut allergy in America, peanuts as well as
peanut butter should not be introduced in the diet until after the
age of two or even later.

Nuts are rich in protein and also a clean source of nourishment,
as they grow on deep-rooted trees and do not contain chemical
residue. Avocados are an appropriate food for infants starting at
six months, and can be mashed with bananas and mixed with
other foods to add a nutritious fat source. The addition of fortified soy milks and tofu, beans, and green vegetables assures complete nutrition for toddlers and children on vegetarian or vegan
diets.

THE REAL QUESTION IS, "CAN AN OMNIVOROUS DIET BE SAFE FOR CHILDREN?"

Clearly the omnivorous diet most children consume today is particularly dangerous to their future health. They eat a diet that receives most of its calories from flour, cheese, oil, and sugar, with negligible fruit and vegetables.

Many American children develop autoimmune illnesses as young adults before heart disease and cancer strike at a later age. Diseases of nutritional ignorance flourish, but they have not been connected to their cause—childhood diets—until now. The amount of animal products consumed and the type of animal products consumed by people including children is a major contributor to the health tragedies that occur later in life. An omnivorous diet with the typical consumption of dairy or meat at every meal is simply foolish.

High dairy fat and animal food consumption in childhood assures unnaturally high levels of hormone promoters that raise our children's blood level of estrogen and testosterone, induce an earlier maturity, and initiate changes that promote adult cancers. One could make an omnivorous diet safer if dairy fat were removed, if one avoided the potential pollutants in fish, if processed food were significantly limited, and if an abundance of produce were consumed.

If you choose a limited amount of animal products to be included in your family's diet, I favor eggs over fish or dairy, because of the potential for transmission of chemicals, mercury, and PCBs in the fish and dairy. Eggs, because they are virtually pollution-free, would be a favored choice over other animal products to add to an otherwise vegan diet.

Therefore, I encourage consumption of a carefully planned vegetarian diet or a carefully planned diet that includes a very small amount of animal products, perhaps 10 percent of total calories or less, rather than the 40 to 60 percent that children eat today. An animal-product-rich omnivorous diet cannot be called healthful.

If one is to utilize animal products in their family's diet they should only choose low-fat or nonfat varieties of dairy products, if they are included in the diet at all. I recommend substituting nuts, seeds, and avocados as the major sources of fat in the diet, instead of dairy fat, oils, and meat.

Fruits, vegetables, avocados, nuts, seeds, beans/legumes, and whole grains are the optimal foods for children. Here are some of the long-term advantages of plant-based diets:

- Vegetarian diets prevent and reduce high blood pressure.[17]

- Cholesterol levels are much lower in vegetarians.[18]

- Cancer rates are much lower in vegetarians.[19]

- Vegetarians are leaner and have less obesity in adulthood.[20]

- Plant-based diets encourage a later menarche, which has been shown to be associated with a reduced risk of prostate and breast cancer.[21]

Both omnivorous and vegetarian diets can be made healthful or harmful, depending on food choices, wise supplementation, and nutritional sophistication. Inclusion of high-nutrient produce, including nuts, seeds, fruits, vegetables, and beans are an essential part of every healthy diet.

RECOMMENDATIONS FOR THE OLDER CHILD OR TEEN

Children possess considerable knowledge and awareness of health education messages.[22] For example, they are well aware of the link between smoking and lung cancer. They have an interest in the reasons why people develop serious illnesses later in life, and they should learn why.

The younger the child, the easier it is to control their food environment, but as they get older, more of the meals are usually eaten away from home, where they are faced with many more food choices.

My children have heard us discuss the relationship between dangerous food and disease causation since they were very young. They were raised with the idea that most people are entirely in the dark about nutritional choices, and that these choices are critical decisions one must make to ensure our happiness and well-being in later life. Children are not stupid, and most will not intentionally harm themselves when taught this important and accurate information about health. Just like the slogan "Say no to drugs and cigarettes," which is taught in school, "Say no to doughnuts, trans fat, processed and smoked meats, and high-fructose corn syrup" can be effectively conveyed. I regularly lecture to teenagers in their school auditoriums, and they almost always ask me intelligent questions that illustrate they want to look good and be healthy. I have frequently had teenagers mention to me that they were either never taught this information or were never taught it in a manner where it made so much sense and had such importance to their future.

COULD DIETARY RESTRICTION OR BECOMING OVERLY CONCERNED ABOUT HEALTHY EATING LEAD TO ANOREXIA NERVOSA?

Some parents fear that adopting dietary guidelines for health and discussing proper weight with their children could lead to anorexia nervosa, particularly in girls. This myth should be dispelled.

While kids on one extreme are getting bigger, a small percentage of children (usually teenage girls) suffer from eating disorders that can cause dangerous malnutrition. Such low calorie and nutrient levels can be harmful and even fatal.

We should not forget that the most common eating disorder is the high-calorie, empty-nutrient diet that most teens eat, leading to an epidemic of overweight adolescents. We know that overweight adolescents have double the chances of heart disease and of dying prematurely of their non-overweight peers.[23] The fear of discussing healthy eating and the importance of a healthy, slim weight should not be discouraged due to an unfounded fear of causing anorexia. We know that anorexia is not the result of teaching and encouraging healthy eating to achieve an ideal weight.

Anorexia nervosa is a serious, potentially life-threatening **mental disorder,** manifesting itself as a failure to maintain a minimal body weight. It occurs predominantly among adolescent females, the majority of whom have underlying depression and anxiety.

This condition stems from psychiatric issues; anorexia is not simply a nutritional problem and its management is difficult and challenging. In many cases the disturbed eating pattern represents a coping effort to manage anger, sadness, and frustration. It is recognized that dysfunctional family dynamics are frequently involved and need to be addressed. This disorder is often preceded by parental psychopathology, maladaptive parenting, childhood maltreatment, and other childhood adversities.[24]

Children or teens with this disorder almost always have distorted misperceptions about their bodies, accompanied by severely restricted dieting and low food intake. The greatly reduced food intake, sometimes feigned as digestive difficulties or food preference, results in nutritional compromise, fatty acid deficiency, and further mental deterioration resulting in depression, irritability, and impaired judgment. Because of its serious and potential life-threatening implications, anorexia should be considered a medical emergency and dealt with accordingly.

Hospital admission is often required, with referral to a hospital psychiatric unit that specializes in the treatment of this disorder. It is important that these individuals receive ongoing counseling, family therapy, psychiatric care, and nutritional guidance and that minimal weight standards are observed.

It is not uncommon for women with eating disorders to follow a vegetarian diet or other restricted eating pattern. However, studies illustrate that health-conscious vegetarians are not at increased risk of anorexia.[25] A person with an eating disorder may choose to follow severely restricted vegetarian diets as a food avoidance excuse, but the diet does not cause anorexia; it is simply a consequence of the eating disorder.

Actually, children who are raised on a wholesome diet are less likely to be stressed about overeating than are those with more abnormal eating patterns. Healthy eating involves more than restricting "bad" food. It involves the consumption of adequate amounts of wholesome foods, including nuts and seeds for essential fat. Children eating healthfully, unlike the anorexic, actually consume large volumes of food and enjoy the ability to eat plenty, while at the same time not having to be overly concerned about their weight. Normal weight is the natural consequence of healthy eating, rather than portion restriction.

Most teens survive on a diet of predominantly junk food. The borderline malnutrition in many teens may predispose them to emotional problems and mental disturbances and may contribute to anorexia nervosa. Healthy eating and healthy parenting will decrease the probability that your child will develop an eating disorder. Anything good—school grades, athletics, good nutrition—can be distorted into something abnormal when combined with a dysfunctional family unit and emotional disturbances. The underlying cause of the malfunction must be addressed to maximize the potential for a full recovery and a healthy life.

A WORKABLE RECIPE FOR TEENAGERS

I have seen hundreds of families with teenage kids radically change their diet as a result of having me as their family physician. They usually begin by watching one of my nutritional videos as a family, followed by a family discussion about it. Another option is to set up family meetings around reading or watching some written materials or sharing some scientific papers about this subject and then discussing it further. A section of this book can be a topic for a family discussion. At the conclusion of every family meeting, they come to a consensus of what they all can do to support one another to make better food choices and how they can incorporate more of this information into their lives.

The Holstroms are a perfect example. Janice Holstrom came to me as a patient first for herself, as she wanted to lose weight, but as she learned about a better way of eating, she was resolute that her husband and children change the way they ate, too. They had a busy lifestyle and picked up fast food at least three nights a week, and all the greasy food in the house was tempting her and sabotaging her good intentions. Her husband, Tom, and their three children resisted any change. The three children (two of them teenagers), Samantha, Trisha, and Carl, were especially unwilling to eat differently. I told Janice to try to have her family watch one of my nutritional videos together. It was better if the teaching about the critical nature of nutrition did not come from her but from me, and would allow them to understand the reasons why Janice became so adamant to eat healthfully and why she wanted the rest of the family to join her. After watching the video, they all agreed to come into my office together to ask me questions.

Trisha, their fifteen-year-old, wanted to know if this way of eating would cure her acne. I assured her that contrary to the prevailing opinion that acne has nothing to do with food, I had scores of teenage patients who cleared or significantly improved their condition with superior nutrition. Superior nutrition results in a healthy complexion without acne, and a low-nutrient diet permits inflammation and the growth of acne-causing bacteria. Acne has everything to do with food.

I taught the children how dangerous it was for their parents to eat the way they had been and enlisted their help so their mom could lower her weight and risk of heart disease and diabetes. Dad had high cholesterol, too.

After some further discussion, they all came to the following agreement: the kids would eat junk food out of the house, and they would remove butter and cheese from the house. They agreed to alternate one vegetarian dinner one night with one non-vegetarian dinner the next. They would limit restaurant food and unhealthy desserts to one per week.

As a family they made a cooking plan, too. Tom would make dinner alone once a week, and Janice would make it twice per week. Two nights of the week both parents would make dinner together. The kids would prepare dinner once a week by themselves and use leftovers, fresh fruit, dried fruit, and nuts to prepare their lunches all by themselves. Once a week they would go out to eat and alternate these excursions so that every other time they would go to a restaurant with a salad bar and vegetable dishes. The other times they would go wherever they chose and could have dessert. They were all pleased with the compromise and felt that they could feel good about their new commitment to health and still have some flexibility so they would not feel deprived.

We talked a little about how to make fruity, healthy ice creams and smoothies, and I gave them some tips on healthy salad dressings and sauces for vegetables. Additionally, I told them what we do in our house: we make a huge pot of vegetable-bean soup once a week and the family all works together to make it and clean up.

When I saw Janice a few months later, surprising to her but not to me was that everyone in the family liked the new recipes and enjoyed eating this way more than their old way. She stated, "Even if this was not so much healthier, the family would still eat this way because they like the new recipes and meals we are making now better than before."

If you have older children, work out a plan that fits your family best. Some people jump in right away; others may prefer to make the change more gradually. Either way, the place to start is the home. The plan can be modified as you go along, but the main thing is for everyone to feel loved, considered, and respected by the others. Your children must know you want them to eat healthy foods because you love them so much and want to protect their future. They will love you back for it.

five

Preparing Healthy Foods That Your Kids Will Love

This chapter contains ten days of suggested menu plans and fifty-seven kid-tested recipes. Not only have these been the recipes and foods that my own kids love to eat, but they have been tested over time with hundreds of children in my medical practice and neighborhood. Food does not have to be unhealthy to taste great. Of course, these recipes are not just for kids. I have taken the healthiest foods in the world and found ways to prepare them to make them delicious and enticing for the entire family. Try many of them and see which ones your kids and family like the best.

I have included many great-tasting vegetarian and vegetable-based dishes designed to make it easy for your children and family to love vegetables.

When you choose an anti-cancer diet style, animal products such as eggs, white-meat turkey, and chicken are viewed as flavorings or condiments used to flavor a vegetable-based meal, rather than as main dishes. Or you may choose a healthy vegan or vegetarian diet for yourself and your family. This chapter contains all those healthy vegan recipes to make eating right easy and fun for you and your children.

CHOOSING A CHILDREN'S CHEWABLE MULTIVITAMIN

- Look for one without vitamin A—vitamin A intake leads to calcium loss in the urine and osteoporosis.[1] We make all the vitamin A we need from the carotenes found in fruits and vegetables.

- A children's supplement should not have more than 2,500 IU of beta-carotene, but even less is better. It is best to receive carotenes from food, not supplements. Studies looking at beta-carotene supplementation show a higher rate of both cancer and heart disease in those supplemented with a high dose of beta-carotene.[2]

- It should contain the full spectrum of minerals.

- It should be free from artificial colors, flavors, and artificial sweeteners.

- It must taste acceptable to your children, as it does no good if your child refuses to take it.

Whether your family is vegetarian or non-vegetarian, I still recommend that everybody in the family take a multivitamin supplement. Not only will our children get additional vitamins and minerals, but most importantly, since plant foods do not contain adequate amounts of vitamin B12, we must make sure children take in enough. Today's vegetation is washed of bacterial and insect residue, removing the B12 that may have been present if the food was collected in the wild. Vitamin D is the sunshine vitamin. It should be considered an important hormone produced by the body from sunshine, but in today's world most people do not get sufficient sunshine to assure optimal levels. Due to depletion of the ozone layer, we avoid the sun more and wear sunscreens to protect us from aging of the skin and skin cancer, so a regular source of vitamin D can be important. Vitamin D is added to cow's milk, but soy milk fortified with vitamin D and vitamin B12 is also a good option. Some orange juices are also fortified with vitamin B12, calcium, and vitamin D and are also a good source of these nutrients, so a multivitamin is not absolutely essential if the diet is otherwise excellent.

Because it is not essential to exclude all animal products from our diet to achieve an anti-cancer diet, I have included a few recipes that demonstrate how animal products can be used in small quantities to flavor a vegetable dish or a soup. The recipes that include animal products are those that contain predominantly nutrient-rich produce, so the small amount of animal products is used to encourage the consumption of more vegetables. The recipes containing some animal products show the ¥ sign. Those desiring to adopt a vegetarian/vegan diet can still utilize those non-vegan dishes by omitting the animal product part of that recipe. Either way, the result is what is commonly referred to as a plant-based diet.

It is easy enough to add small strips of white-meat turkey or chicken to add texture and flavor to a soup or vegetable dish. One ounce per person is sufficient. The crucial distinction between this new anti-cancer way of eating, compared to the traditional way of serving a slab of animal meat on a plate, is that one traditional serving of animal product is split up in the vegetable dish or soup and used for the entire family for a few nights. In other words, animal products become condiments, not main dishes. In that manner the diet retains the benefits of a plant-based vegetarian diet without having to exclude animal products entirely.

Of course, many will choose to follow a totally vegetarian or

vegan diet such as recommended by the famous physician and author Dr. Benjamin Spock. Dr. Spock was our nation's most trusted
pediatrician and bestselling author of all time. His most recent and
updated book advocated a vegetarian diet for children and their parents for many of the reasons stated in this book. He wanted to protect children against the development of later life diseases, which
we now know are largely avoidable. He was a courageous advocate
on behalf of children and was not afraid to take a stance contrary to
the establishment. Unfortunately, mainstream views are frequently
ten to twenty years behind the times, and attempt to conform to
politically and socially accepted standards.

TEN SUPER FOODS TO USE IN YOUR
RECIPES AND MENUS

Avocados are a clean, healthy source of healthy fatty acids. They
are rich in cholesterol-lowering phytosterols and high in the powerful anti-oxidant glutathione. Avocados are a healthy anti-cancer
food. Use it in place of butter, mash it with bananas for young children, and use it in lots of avocado-based dressings and dips.

Blueberries/Blackberries These darkly colored berries are packed
with tannins, anthocyanidins, flavonoids, polyphenols, and proanth-
cyanidins that have been linked to prevention and reversal of age-
related mental decline. They also have powerful anti-cancer effects.
Use frozen organic berries in the winter when fresh ones are not
available.

Cantaloupes are another vitamin powerhouse. With only 56 calories a cup, one gets a huge amount of vitamin C and beta-carotene
as well as folate, potassium, fiber, thiamin, niacin, pantothenic acid,
and vitamin B6. We take half a cantaloupe and blend it with one
cup of ice cubes and a few dates to make a frothy cantaloupe slush;
the kids love it.

Carrots/Beets are colorful root crops that add beauty and flavor to dishes. Shredded raw in salads, cooked, or in soups, they are high in fiber and antioxidant compounds such as caratonoids and beta-cyanin, a powerful cancer protective agent found to inhibit cell mutations. In our house we frequently add fresh-squeezed carrot and beet juice to our soup recipes.

Flax Seeds are rich in lignans and omega-3 fatty acids, and scientific studies have confirmed that flax seeds have a positive influence on everything from cholesterol levels and constipation to cancer and heart disease. Use ground flax seeds in oatmeal, or add them to whipped frozen bananas, stewed apples, and cinnamon and nut balls. Keep in mind that the scientifically documented benefits from flax seeds come from raw, ground flax seed, not flax seed oil.

Green Lettuce is exceptionally low in calories, but contains an abundance of phytonutrients, plant proteins, vitamins, minerals, and fiber. Eat salad with lettuce every day. Our children like to eat lettuce leaves plain, and we always leave some washed leaves of romaine lettuce in a bowl for them to snack on.

Kale is a fantastic high-nutrient green vegetable to add to soups and to serve chopped. My children devour the stuff. We serve steamed and chopped kale with a cashew nut cream sauce.

Sesame Seeds are one of the most mineral-rich foods in the world and a potent source of calcium, magnesium, copper, iron, manganese, zinc, vitamins, and fiber. They are also rich in anti-cancer lignans that are uniquely found in sesame seeds alone. Grind some unhulled sesame seeds into a powder to sprinkle on salads and vegetables. Toast lightly and mix with eggplant, chickpeas, scallions, and garlic for a healthy and delicious dip.

Strawberries are high in folic acid, flavonoids, iron, and vitamin C. They provide a good source of dietary fiber and potassium yet contain only 60 calories per cup. Use strawberries and frozen strawberries frequently. We serve a desert of strawberries and whipped cream for the kids. The creamy whipped cream is made by blending raw macadamia nuts with a few dates and soy milk until smooth. We also add frozen strawberries to our whipped frozen bananas. Try a fruit smoothie by blending together a banana, orange juice, and frozen strawberries.

Tomatoes have been a hot topic in recent years because their consumption has been linked to dramatic reduction in the incidence of common cancers. One of tomatoes' heavily investigated anti-cancer phytochemicals is lycopene, which has been shown to be protective against cancer, including prostate cancer, breast cancer, endometrial cancer, lung cancer, and colorectal cancers.

WHAT IS ON THE MAIN MENU?

These recipes are especially designed to include dishes that utilize flax seeds, blueberries, greens, nuts, and other special disease-fighting foods that are so beneficial to our long-term health. There is a huge variety of foods and dishes to choose from. You can incorporate recipes utilizing the healthiest parts of cuisines from all over the world, including Japanese, Chinese, Mediterranean, and Italian. Get set for a taste adventure as we explore this new way of eating using ideas from all over the globe. Healthy eating does not have to be boring, and you can learn to please the palate of the strongest skeptic.

This chapter contains ten days of suggested menu plans utilizing the recipes that follow. Try the ones you think your family will like the best and then make a two-week plan for your house. You will probably repeat many of the recipes that you like best more than once in a ten-day period. In my house we generally make a large enough quantity so we eat leftovers the next day, and our soups may last for three to four days. Cooking in large quantities saves work, so we only prepare time-consuming meals three days a week. Experiment with what works best in your house. That way you can shop in advance for the food and ingredients you need each week and it will become easier as you plan out the days you shop, what you purchase, and the time needed to set aside for food preparation.

Let me know how you do and how your children like the new foods. Many more great recipes are included in *Eat to Live,* my longevity and weight loss book, designed for adults who want to lose weight in the healthiest manner possible, and there are hundreds of more recipes available on my Web site, drfuhrman.com, as well. If you design some of your own special healthy recipes, send them my way, too, so I can share them with my online community of health seekers.

GET READY, GET SET, COOK

Keep in mind that most of the foods your children and family consume can be simple fruits, raw vegetables, and nuts that require no preparation. Always keep lots of fresh fruit and raw vegetables such as sliced peppers, celery, cherry tomatoes, okra, raw string beans, English peas, and snow pea pods available and left out in bowls on the kitchen table at all times, so the children can grab and snack on them as they please. These vegetables are fine to leave unrefrigerated for a few days, and you will be surprised at how the raw vegetables and raw nuts slowly disappear. Instead of flowers to decorate your tables, use bowls of seasonal fresh fruit. It is fine for your children to forage during the day and eat less at mealtimes. Offer an array of healthful food and let them control their own intake. Over time you will realize you do not need to cook and prepare a complete array of foods at dinner. A salad, one cooked main dish, and a simple fruit-based dessert are sufficient.

Steaming vegetables and making soups is called water-based cooking. Water-based cooking is the preferred way to cook because you can avoid cancer-causing acrylamides that are created when foods are browned by baking or frying.

Never eat browned or overly cooked food. Burnt food forms harmful compounds. If by accident something is overcooked and browned, discard it. Avoid fried food and food sautéed in oil. Most of the baked recipes that follow are cooked at a very low heat, and they can be cooked at an even lower heat by leaving the oven door ajar with a little crack for hot air to escape. Experiment with low-heat cooking to prevent nutritional damage to the food and the formation of dangerous heat-generated compounds.

All the recipes in this book are dairy-free. Because I consider dairy fat dangerous and since so many children are lactose-intolerant, these recipes show you how to make calcium-rich and nutrient-rich meals without dairy. Soy milk is available fortified with vitamin D and calcium, and I find it very useful for making delicious smoothies and fruit-based desserts. There are many brands to pick from that all taste slightly different. It is easy to find one that suits your taste and the taste preferences of your child.

You will need a good food processor or quality blender for many of the recipes. I recommend owning a centrifugal juicer, an orange juicer, and a food processor or high-quality blending machine. The blenders that contain a plunger to stir and force the food down into the blades are helpful for making fruit-based sorbets, sauces, and dressings.

ELEVEN HOT TIPS FOR YOUR KITCHEN MAKEOVER

1. Remove temptation. Go through your kitchen removing from your cupboard all the junk food and processed food and dump it. Clean out your freezer, too, while you are at it.

2. Make a sign for the refrigerator listing what foods are inside, such as split pea soup, washed grapes, apple surprise,

and eggplant dip. Make it easy for the family to find out what healthy foods are available. Have fun. Consider posting an advertisement on a bulletin board with larger letters and colorful stars and hearts for the dish you are encouraging for the day. Be flashy and creative. It works.

3. Keep a bowl of ready-to-eat raw fruits and vegetables on your kitchen counter. Include cherry tomatoes, raw string beans, raw peeled carrot slices, snow pea pods, grapes, strawberries, melon cubes, and cut pineapple. Putting a healthy (nut-based) dip near the veggies is also a great idea.

4. Make several ears of steamed corn on the cob and keep them cold in the fridge for fast meals on the go. Meals and snacks that are easy to find, grab, and run with make it easy for your family to make healthy choices. Air-popped popcorn lightly sprayed with olive oil from a mist spray bottle and sprinkled with nutritional yeast is a tasty snack.

5. Soak dried fruits, such as unsulphered sun-dried apricots or mangoes, in a little unsweetened soy milk, or dried pineapple in a little orange juice, to use as natural sweeteners to add when whipping frozen fruit in the blender or food processor to make delicious natural sorbets for dessert the next day. Keep sun-dried tomatoes soaking in a plastic bag with a little water, too, to add cut up to make salads or vegetable dishes.

6. Make extra servings of oatmeal mixed with apples and cinnamon and keep the leftovers in the refrigerator for a quick breakfast on the go.

7. Stock your cupboard with raisins, currents, dates, seeds, and nuts. Keep plenty of frozen vegetables and fruits in your freezer.

8. Make lots of trail mix packets for your family. Put together some "grab-and-go" minibags of raisins and diced dried apples with nuts and seeds.

9. Buy healthy breads that are 100 percent whole grain, coarsely ground, and low in salt.

10. Remove butter and conventional margarine and instead use only the trans-fat-free healthy spreads.

11. Cut up a fresh pineapple or a melon, or juice or peel enough fresh oranges, so all can have some fresh fruit or fresh juice every morning.

PACKING A LUNCH FOR SCHOOL

One main message of this book is to avoid the typical school lunch of luncheon meats and cheese. Typical school lunches are greasy, salty, and of poor nutritional quality. Lots of the great-tasting, healthful recipes in this chapter include soups, puddings, and salads, so make sure you have a small container with a tight lid that your child can open and bring back home in her knapsack or book bag daily. Kids like soup cold, even when not at school, so you don't have to worry about rewarming it. If your child doesn't bring home the containers you may want to buy some small disposable plastic ones.

Some children are happy to eat healthfully, but when it comes to school lunch they don't want to look different from the other kids. Packing fresh fruit and a healthy bread with some nut butter and an unsweetened fruit spread can be a quick option. Try adding banana slices for a healthy nut butter sandwich. My children love raw cashew nut butter. If using peanut butter, purchase a brand without salt and other additives. My daughters also like to take peeled oranges or apple slices with their lunch. We cut the apple into four sections around the core, most of the way through, keeping the apple intact, and then wrap it in silver foil. This way it stays fresh, without discoloration, and they can easily separate it into slices.

Whole-wheat pita pockets are a great option for a bag lunch. Any of your child's favorite healthy salad dressings can be used to line the pita, which is then stuffed with a slice of tomato and salad. You can fill them with almost anything, including dinner leftovers, bean and mushroom burgers, salad, avocado hummus, rice, potato salad, or fruit. Many of the recipes below can be used as is or stuffed into a whole-wheat pita and wrapped in foil. My kids love avocado, tomato, and shredded lettuce with the Hot Russian Dressing (recipe below) stuffed into a pita. If making pitas or sandwiches with sprouts and tomatoes, make a great healthy spread by mashing avocado with some mustard. Always pack some fruit with their lunch—add some cut-up pineapple, a peeled orange, a banana, or any fruit in season.

THE RECIPES MAY MENTION:

Vita-Mix is an expensive, high-powered blender with a plunger that facilitates the making of soups, dressings, sauces, and smoothies. It is worth the investment.

VegeBase is an instant vegetable soup mix that can be added to soups or vegetable dishes as a flavoring.

Mrs. Dash is a no-salt-added blend of spices for vegetable dishes and soups. It comes in various flavors.

Braggs Liquid Amino's is a soybean-based liquid that adds a mild soy sauce–like flavor to vegetables, but is much lower in sodium than traditional soy sauces.

THE RECIPES

....

SOUPS
Cabbage Raisin Soup
Carrot Cream Soup
Peachy Leek Soup
Split Pea and Tofu Dog
Tomato Tornado
Vegetable Pea/Bean Soup

SALADS AND DRESSINGS
Dr. Flax's Sesame Seasoning
Green Banana Power Blended Salad
Hot Russian Dressing
Orange Cashew Dressing
Patriotic Salad
Pecan Maple Salad

VEGETABLES/BEANS AND MAIN DISHES
Apricot Brown Rice
Avocadole Guacamole
British Baked Tofu
Broccoli with Garlic
California Creamed Kale
Chocolaty Lentils
Eggplant Sicilian
Healthy Potato Fries
Lettuce Tasty Rolls
Mild Bean Chutney
Oriental Chicken and Broccoli ¥
Purple Potato Salad ¥

Quick Soy Cheese Pita Pizza

Quinoa and Nut Loaf

Red-Hot Hummus

Squash Fantasia

St. Patty's Peanut Butter and Date Jelly Sandwich

String Beans and Almond Dust

Sushi for Your Tootsie

Sweet Potato Pie with Secret Walnuts

Teriyaki Chicken Coleslaw ¥

Tofu Pizza Slices

Quinoa in Color

Vegetable Lasagna

Veggie Meat Loaf ¥

Wild Rice and Broccoli

FRUIT DISHES/BREAKFAST FOODS AND DESSERTS

Almond Carob Fudge

Apple Pecan Pudding

Apple Walnut Surprise

Baked Apple with Cashew Raisin Cream Sauce

Banana Nut Cookies

Banana/Pineapple Sorbet

Blueberry and Flax Yogurt

Cantaloupe Slush

Carob-Avocado Cream Pie

Date Nut Pop'ems

Flax/Oatmeal Bars

Fuhrman Fudgsicles

Peach Sorbet

Rice Pudding with Banana/Apricot Sauce

Soy Milk Fruit Smoothies

Tuttie Fruitie Pita Sandwich

Vanilla-Carob Fudge
Whipped Banana Freeze
Whipped Cream and Strawberries

SOUPS

....

CABBAGE RAISIN SOUP
Serves 4–6

3 tablespoons lemon juice
3 large onions, chopped
¼ cup split peas
¼ cup pearl barley
1 head of green cabbage, large chunks
1 cup raisins or currents
1 cup chopped walnuts
1 cup unsweetened soy milk
2 cups fresh-squeezed apple juice
4 cups water
2 cups chopped carrots
1 teaspoon oregano
2 tablespoons dehydrated vegetable soup mix such as VegeBase
1 teaspoon Mrs. Dash

Blend the raisins with two cups of water in a good blender, food processor, or Vita-Mix until smooth and creamy. Add the liquefied raisins and the rest of the ingredients together in the pot and cook on a very low flame. Leave the cabbage in large chunks. When the cabbage is soft remove it from the soup with tongs and blend it into the soup liquid in the blender or Vita-Mix again. Add it back to the soup and continue cooking in a covered pot on a low flame another hour until done.

CARROT CREAM SOUP

Serves 4–6

20 carrots, washed, peeled, and cut into large chunks

2 potatoes, peeled and cut into large chunks

3 onions, peeled and chopped

2 cups soy milk

2 cups water

1 small zucchini, sliced

1 tablespoon minced fresh ginger root (optional)

2 cloves garlic

1 tablespoon dehydrated vegetable instant soup mix or
   VegeBase

¼ cup raw cashews

¼ cup raw almonds

Make this quick, thick, and creamy soup by adding all the ingredients except the nuts to a pot and simmer on low heat for 20 minutes. Then puree the cooked soup with the nuts in a food processor or good blender until smooth.

PEACHY LEEK SOUP

Serves 4

2 cups dried peaches (soaked in 1 cup of water overnight)

1-pound bag frozen peaches

½ cup lentils

4 large onions

2 leek stalks, split and washed

2 pounds carrots, juiced

4-ounce bag of spinach

4 cups water

Blend the frozen peaches into the water until smooth and add to a large, covered soup pot.

Chop the soaked dried peaches into small chunks and place in the soup pot with the soaking water, set on a low flame. Add the lentils, chopped onions, and leeks. Take all the carrot juice and blend the raw spinach into it in a blender, food processor, or Vita-Mix and then add to the pot. Take the soft cooked leeks out of the soup pot and blend until smooth with the soup liquid and pour back into the pot. Simmer on a low flame in a covered pot another 30 minutes.

SPLIT PEA AND TOFU DOG
Serves 4–6

1 cup fresh or frozen carrot juice
1 cup fresh or frozen celery juice
1 cup soy milk
2 cups water
2 cups dry split peas
2 cups chopped onions
3 cloves minced garlic
1 tablespoon Mrs. Dash
1 tablespoon minced rosemary
3 tofu hot dogs, sliced into small slices

Add all the dry ingredients into the liquid portion and simmer for 45 minutes.

TOMATO TORNADO
Serves 2

½ cup pinto beans
4 cups fresh tomato, chopped

2 apples, cored

1 onion, sliced

1 cup unsweetened soy milk

½ cup corn kernels

3 tablespoons tomato paste

1 tablespoon VegeBase Instant Soup Mix, or another dried
　　vegetable soup base

1 tablespoon apple cider vinegar or raisin vinegar.

Blend pinto beans, 2 tomatoes, apples, onion, and soy milk in food processor or blender. Add 2 chopped tomatoes, corn, tomato paste, VegeBase, and vinegar. Simmer on low heat until tomatoes are soft.

VEGETABLE PEA/BEAN SOUP

Serves 6

2 cups carrot juice

2 cups celery juice

4 cups water

4 cups kale, chopped

8 carrots, chopped

6 onions, finely chopped

8 tomatoes, finely chopped, retain all juice

½ cup dried split peas

½ cup mixed dried soup beans

5 tablespoons Powered Vegetable Soup Mix or VegeBase

1 tablespoon Mrs. Dash Table Blend

Combine all ingredients and simmer on low heat for 90 minutes.

SALADS AND DRESSINGS

....

DR. FLAX'S SESAME SEASONING
1 tablespoon ground flax seeds
1 tablespoon ground unhulled raw sesame seeds
1 teaspoon onion flakes
½ teaspoon garlic powder
2 tablespoons VegeBase

Use a coffee grinder or Vita-Mix to grind the flax and sesame seeds. Flax seeds can also be purchased already ground. Mix all the ingredients together and put in a shaker with wide holes. Use liberally on vegetables and soups instead of salt and other seasonings. Store in refrigerator when not in use.

GREEN BANANA POWER BLENDED SALAD
Serves 2

2–3 ounces washed baby spinach
3–4 ounces washed romaine lettuce
1 banana
½ avocado
5 medjool dates
1 tablespoon black fig vinegar (optional)

Blend well into a smooth pudding-like consistency in the food processor, the Vita-Mix, or a powerful blender by shoving the lettuce down into the blades with a cucumber or carrot used as a plunging tool. Blending raw greens until smooth greatly increases the absorption of nutrients from our digestive tract, delivering a powerful nutrient punch.

HOT RUSSIAN DRESSING
Serves 4–6

1 small (4-ounce) can tomato paste
4 tablespoons raw almond butter
¼ teaspoon chili powder
¼ cup soy milk
3 tablespoons ketchup

Blend all ingredients together. Works well as a sauce for steamed leafy greens; as a condiment spread for lettuce, tomato, and avocado pita pocket sandwiches; and as a salad dressing.

ORANGE CASHEW DRESSING
Serves 4–6

2 peeled navel oranges
¼ cup orange juice
¼ cup raw cashews
2 tablespoons of blood orange vinegar or pear vinegar

Blend ingredients until silky smooth. Use liberally on salad or as vegetable dip.

PATRIOTIC SALAD
Serves 1

½ cup soy milk
1 banana
8–12 leaves of romaine lettuce
1 cup fresh or frozen blueberries
1 cup fresh or frozen strawberries

Blend the soy milk and banana together. Shred the lettuce, mix with the fruit, and pour the banana-soy mixture over it.

PECAN MAPLE SALAD
Serves 4–6

½ cup chopped pecans
½ cup regular (original) soy milk
1½ teaspoons cinnamon
2 medjool dates
2 tablespoons of pure maple syrup
2 tablespoons spicy pecan vinegar (optional)

Mix in blender half the chopped pecans with the other ingredients. Then when creamy take out of the blender and add the rest of the pecans so the dressing remains lumpy, with some crunch. Pour over baby romaine lettuce or spinach for that soft but crunchy salad. It is also good with chunks of pear mixed in.

VEGETABLES/BEANS AND MAIN DISHES

....

APRICOT BROWN RICE
Serves 4–6

2 cups brown rice
¼ teaspoon ground cumin
½ teaspoon coriander
½ teaspoon cinnamon
1 cup dried apricots (organic sun-dried)
3 cups water
½ cup sunflower seeds

Cook brown rice, spices, and dried apricots with 3 cups water on low heat for 35 minutes. Add sunflower seeds and simmer for 10 more minutes. Remove from flame. Toss with one tablespoon flax seed oil and serve.

AVOCADOLE GUACAMOLE
Serves 4–6

2 avocados
2 tomatoes
2 tablespoons tomato paste
2 tablespoons onion flakes
½ cup currents or raisins
1 tablespoon coriander leaves
2 tablespoons chopped parsley
juice of ½ lemon
1 tablespoon date sugar

In a quality blender or food processor, blend all ingredients until smooth. Serve as a dip for vegetables or toasted pita, or serve over brown rice or cut-up baked or steamed potato chunks.

BRITISH BAKED TOFU
Serves 4–6

2 blocks firm tofu
4 cloves garlic
1 yellow onion
½ teaspoon chili powder
¼ cup apple cider vinegar

Cut each block of firm tofu into 16 strips. Divide it into four slices first, and then make four tofu strips out of every slice. Blend together the remaining ingredients, adding just enough water to cover the tofu strips to marinate them overnight. Bake in the oven for 200 degrees for two hours, until tofu yellows and hardens. Great as snacks and with school lunches, or placed on whole-grain sandwiches with lettuce, tomato, and Hot Russian Dressing.

BROCCOLI WITH GARLIC
Serves 4–6

2 large bunches of broccoli or three boxes of frozen broccoli
4 cloves garlic, pressed or minced
1 tablespoon Dijon-style mustard
1 tablespoon olive oil

Steam broccoli for 5 to 7 minutes or defrost frozen broccoli. Remove from heat and cut up into pieces in large salad bowl. Mix the oil, garlic, and mustard together and toss the broccoli with the mixture. Return to steamer to cook for another 5 minutes. The dressing in this recipe is delicious on other green vegetables as well. Try it with okra, asparagus, green beans, and string beans.

CALIFORNIA CREAMED KALE
Serves 4–6

2 pounds raw kale
½ cup raw cashew nuts
½ cup soy milk
2 tablespoons onion flakes
1 tablespoon VegeBase Instant Soup Mix

Remove the thick bottom of the stems from the kale and place the leaves in a large pot with steamer. Steam 10 minutes, until soft. Remove from steamer, placing in wooden chopping bowl. Press the kale together in the bowl with a dish towel and tilt over the sink to remove some of the excess water.

Add the remaining ingredients to the blender and blend until smooth. Chop the kale, mixing it with the cream sauce as you chop.

CHOCOLATY LENTILS

Serves 2–3

3 pitted dates
¼ cup soy milk
1 tablespoon raw carob powder (optional)
1 can unsalted lentils or lentils with bay leaves
1 cup chopped plum tomatoes

Blend dates with soy milk and carob to make cream sauce, then mix it well with the can of lentils and the chopped tomatoes.

EGGPLANT SICILIAN

Serves 4–6

2 egg whites
¼ cup soy milk
½ cup Italian seasoned whole-wheat bread crumbs
½ cup whole-wheat flour
3 large onions
2 large firm eggplants
1 cup no-salt tomato sauce
4 ounces soy cheese

Whip the egg whites together with the soy milk. Mix the bread crumbs together with the flour. Slice the onions into very thin onion patties and slice the eggplant into ¼-inch patties. Layer a baking pan with the thin onion slices. Dip the eggplant into the egg mixture and then in the flour mix to lightly bread and place on top of the onion. Place another thin slice of onion on top of the eggplant and put a thin coating of tomato sauce on top, then add another layer of eggplant on top. Add one more thin layer of tomato sauce and then cover with a thin sliver of soy cheese, cut with a cheese slicer, on the top. Bake in the oven at 250 degrees for 40 minutes. You can also use this for school lunches by using it as a stuffing for a whole-wheat pita.

HEALTHY POTATO FRIES
Serves 3–4

6 white potatoes, scalloped or cut into strips
2 cups apple juice
Olive oil in spray bottle

Mix the potatoes well with the apple juice and let sit for 5 minutes. Toss again and pour off the juice, leaving the wet slices of potato. Spray a light coating of olive oil on a nonstick baking tray and spread out the potatoes. Add a few more sprays of the oil over the top of the potatoes and bake in the oven at 325 degrees for 15 minutes on one side and 7 minutes on the other.

LETTUCE TASTY ROLLS
Serves 2–4

½ cup almond butter
¼ cup tomato paste

pinch of chili powder

2 cups shredded carrots

¼ cup shredded red onion

1 diced tomato

1 diced red pepper

1 teaspoon chopped basil

12 large leaves of romaine with center white stalk cut out

Mash the almond butter with the tomato paste and chili powder and spread the mixture thinly onto each lettuce leaf. Mix all the shredded and diced vegetables together and sprinkle over each leaf. Roll up the leaves, using toothpicks to hold them together. Option: use avocado instead of almond butter.

MILD BEAN CHUTNEY

Serves 4–6

1 cup diced tomatoes

1 cup shredded green cabbage

1 cup shredded carrots

1 cup diced green peppers

½ lemon

½ cup diced red onions

1 cup frozen corn, defrosted

1 cup chickpeas

1 cup frozen green peas, defrosted

1 teaspoon cumin

1 tablespoon wine vinegar or raisin vinegar

1 teaspoon Mrs. Dash

1 teaspoon garlic powder

1 cup red kidney beans

1 cup black beans

Add the tomatoes to a small covered pot and steam the shredded cabbage, carrots, and green peppers for only 5 minutes on the lowest flame possible in the pot. Stir in juice of ½ lemon and the diced red onions, corn, peas, spices, and beans.

Serve cold on top of shredded lettuce.

ORIENTAL CHICKEN AND BROCCOLI ¥
Serves 4–6

6 ounces skinless chicken breast
32 ounces fresh broccoli
1 can water chestnuts
1 can baby corn
1 cup pearl ear mushrooms
1 tablespoon sesame oil
1 egg white
1 tablespoon date sugar
1 tablespoon cornstarch
3 tablespoons chunky pineapple with juice
1 teaspoon Bragg's Liquid Aminos

Place chicken in small steamer and steam for 25 minutes, then dice into small chunks. Steam broccoli in big pot for 15 minutes. Add the water chestnuts, baby corn, and small mushrooms and steam for 5 minutes more.

Whip the sesame oil with the egg white, then fold in the date sugar, cornstarch, pineapple with juice, and Bragg's Liquid Aminos. On low heat mix and simmer for 3 minutes.

Mix all ingredients together and toss. This recipe gives 10 ounces of vegetables per person with only 1.5 ounces of chicken as a flavoring. It is also good without the chicken.

PURPLE POTATO SALAD ¥
Serves 4–6

5 pounds of potatoes, peeled
3 large onions, chopped
1 tablespoon olive oil
6 cups shredded red cabbage (about ½ cabbage)
6 hard-boiled eggs, discard 3 yolks
3 tablespoons canola oil mayonnaise
3 tablespoons soy milk
½ cup chopped scallions
1 cup chopped celery

Steam potatoes until soft, then refrigerate. Sautée onions in nonstick pan with a thin coating of olive oil for 3 minutes and add cabbage on top. Cover pan with tight lid and cook onion-cabbage mixture for an additional 5 minutes, stirring occasionally. It is okay if the cabbage is cooked unevenly, with some parts well cooked and other parts not.

Mix the 3 hard-boiled egg whites with the mayo and soy milk with a fork and mash together. Place the scallions, celery, potatoes, remaining 3 hardboiled eggs, and potatoes in a bowl and chop, mixing as you chop. Fold in the sautéed onions and cabbages as you mix everything together, chill, and serve.

QUICK SOY CHEESE PITA PIZZA
Serves 4

4 large whole-wheat pitas
1 cup no-salt tomato sauce
½ cup chopped mushrooms

½ cup chopped red onions

10 ounces frozen broccoli florets, thawed and chopped fine

1 cup white soy cheese

Slice edges of pita and separate to make 8 pita pizzas. Lay flat on baking tray and spoon on the tomato sauce. Sprinkle evenly with the mushrooms, onions, and broccoli and cover with a light application of shredded soy cheese. Bake on a low temperature (200 degrees) in the oven for 15 minutes.

QUINOA AND NUT LOAF
Serves 4

1 cup quinoa

1 cup chopped onions

3 tablespoons tomato paste

2 tablespoons chopped parsley

½ cup diced celery

½ cup diced red peppers

½ cup pine nuts

½ cup chopped filberts

1 teaspoon Mrs. Dash Italian seasoning

1 teaspoon nutritional or brewer's yeast

pinch of garlic powder

Cook the quinoa and onion in two cups water and let simmer in a covered pot on a low flame for 15 minutes.

In a separate bowl put the tomato paste, parsley, celery, peppers, nuts, and seasonings and mix well. Mix well with the quinoa/onion mix and place in glass loaf dish in the oven for 30 minutes at 200 degrees. Many like this delicious main dish with a tomato sauce.

RED-HOT HUMMUS

Serves 4

1 cup canned (unsalted) chickpeas
3 tablespoons unhulled raw sesame seeds
2 tablespoons lemon
½ red onion, chopped
2 tablespoons tomato paste
pinch of chili powder to taste

Blend ingredients in blender or food processor until creamy. If necessary, add a small amount of water to assist in blending. Serve as dip or sandwich spread with lettuce, tomatoes, and sprouts.

SQUASH FANTASIA

Serves 4–8

1 cup dried apricots
½ cup raisins or currants
1 cup orange juice
4 butternut squashes
¼ cup raw sunflower seeds
¼ cup raw pumpkin seeds

Soak dried apricots and raisins in orange juice overnight. Cut squash in half, scoop out seed bowl, and remove seeds. Place in baking dish with ¼ inch of water at the bottom and cover lightly with silver foil. Bake in oven at 300 degrees for 30 minutes. Meanwhile, chop apricots and raisins in food processor or hand chopper. Chop sunflower seeds and pumpkin seeds in food processor or hand chopper. Mix the seeds and moist dried fruits together. Remove the squash from the oven and scoop the seed-fruit mix into the bowl of the squash. Add a little more orange juice if necessary to fill the bowl. Bake for 15 more minutes. Remove the squash from oven and serve as is, or for children mash the squash, mixing it with the fruit/nut mix before serving.

ST. PATTY'S PEANUT BUTTER AND DATE JELLY SANDWICH
Serves 4

1 cup frozen peas, thawed
¼ cup unsalted peanut butter
whole-grain bread
2 medjool dates
½ cup dried apricots or mangoes
½ cup soy milk

Mash peas with fork and mix and mash well with peanut butter. Spread on coarse whole grain bread with date jelly. Date jelly is made by mashing 2 medjool dates with dried apricots or dried mangoes that have been soaked overnight in soy milk.

STRING BEANS AND ALMOND DUST
Serves 4

1 cup slivered almonds
¼ cup unhulled sesame seeds
2 pounds string beans with top stems cut off
½ teaspoon flax oil
½ teaspoon olive oil

Take half of the slivered almonds and sesame seeds and grind into powder in coffee grinder, food processor, or Vita-Mix. Lay out the other half of the nuts in pan in toaster oven and lightly toast on lowest setting possible. Steam the string beans and hand-toss with flax oil and olive oil. Mix in the toasted nut dust and sprinkle the toasted nuts on top of each serving.

SUSHI FOR YOUR TOOTSIE
Serves 4

½ cup short-grain brown rice
4 sheets of seaweed sushi wrap (purchase in health food store
   or oriental market)
1 tablespoon mustard
1 tablespoon canola mayo
1 teaspoon onion flakes
¼ cup raw unhulled sesame seeds
½ cup shredded carrots
1 avocado, sliced thin

Soak the rice in 2 cups water for one hour, then bring to boil on as low a heat as possible in a covered pot and do not remove the cover to look at or stir the rice. Lower the heat even more in 5 minutes when boiling lightly to cook the rice as slowly as possible for another 15 minutes. Then let the rice sit for another 30 minutes, off the flame, without taking off the cover. This will make the rice soft and sticky to use in the sushi.

Lay the seaweed sheets on a piece of plastic wrap and then spread rice smoothly to about ¼ inch thick with back of spoon evenly over the seaweed. Brush on a very thin coating of mustard and mayo mixed together and then sprinkle it with some onion flakes and the raw unhulled sesame seeds that have been toasted lightly in a pan. Lay a strip of shredded carrots and avocado along one end.

Begin rolling by lifting plastic under seaweed roll and pressing ingredients with fingers. Roll up carefully. Repeat using all ingredients to make 4 rolls. Cut each roll crosswise into 6 to 8 equal slices. Best refrigerated and eaten cold.

SWEET POTATO PIE WITH SECRET WALNUTS
Serves 6–8

6 sweet potatoes
2 peeled navel oranges
¼ cup orange juice
2 tablespoons date sugar
1 cup walnut halves
1 15-ounce can unsweetened pineapple rings

Bake sweet potatoes 70 minutes, until soft. Remove from oven and remove skin and any browned area. Blend oranges, juice, date sugar, and walnuts together in blender or food processor and mix or process in the sweet potato. Spoon out into glass baking dish, place pineapple rings on top, and bake for another 10 minutes at 300 degrees.

TERIYAKI CHICKEN COLESLAW ¥
Serves 4

1 cup raisins
2 white potatoes, boiled
½ cup soy milk
2 tablespoons onion flakes
1 tablespoon olive oil
1 tablespoon flax seed oil
1 tablespoon VegeBase
1 teaspoon Mrs. Dash seasoning

½ green cabbage, shredded
1 cup snow pea pods, shredded
6 ounces chicken breast, cooked and shredded

Mix and mash white potatoes, soy milk, onion flakes, and oil and seasonings to form a thick sauce. Mix thoroughly with the shredded vegetables, raisins, and chicken. Serve chilled.

TOFU PIZZA SLICES
Serves 4

2 blocks of firm tofu
1 jar unsalted tomato sauce

Slice the tofu into very thin, flat slices and lay over thin wire rack. Pour or spoon lots of tomato sauce on each slice and bake at 250 degrees for 2 hours.

QUINOA IN COLOR
Serves 4

1 cup rinsed quinoa
2 cups water
¼ cup red peppers, chopped
¼ cup green peppers, chopped
¼ cup yellow peppers, chopped
¼ cup orange peppers, chopped
¼ cup red onions, chopped
¼ cup carrots, chopped
2 cloves garlic, chopped
½ teaspoon chili powder
1 can (16 ounces) organic pinto or adzuki beans

Mix all ingredients in a pot, except the beans. Bring to a boil and then turn down heat to simmer for about 15 minutes, until most of the liquid is absorbed. Turn off heat and add the can of beans.

VEGETABLE LASAGNA
Serves 4

1 pound firm tofu
¼ cup lemon juice
¼ cup sesame tahini
¼ cup shredded coconut
¼ cup nutritional yeast
2 tablespoons chopped parsley
2 cups diced carrots
1 medium zucchini
1 medium yellow squash
1 bunch of broccoli, chopped
1 cup unsalted tomato sauce
1 tablespoon oregano
1 tablespoon Italian seasoning
1 cup chopped scallions
1 package whole-wheat lasagna noodles, boiled per package
    instructions
1 cup shredded soy cheese

Blend the tofu, lemon juice, tahini, shredded coconut, nutritional yeast, and parsley in a food processor and put aside. Blend all the vegetables with the tomato sauce and the oregano, Italian seasoning, and scallions to make a thick veggie paste. Place a small amount of sauce in the bottom of a large casserole pan. Make layers of cooked lasagna noodles by spreading tofu mixture on top of the noodles, then another layer of noodles, and then the veggie mix. Put the last layer of noodles on top, sprinkle the shredded soy cheese on the top, cover the top of the dish, and bake in the oven at 350 degrees for 40 minutes.

VEGGIE MEAT LOAF ¥
Serves 4

The same recipe can be made vegan, without the meat, for a different flavor.

1 cup sunflower seeds
1 cup almonds
1 cup chopped carrots
2 garlic cloves
1 red onion
½ cup finely chopped parsley
1 cup chopped red pepper
1 cup chopped celery
6 ounces lean steak, ground
1 tomato
1 tablespoon tomato paste
½ teaspoon oregano
1 teaspoon chopped basil
¼ teaspoon black pepper
¼ teaspoon chili powder
1 head of lettuce, shredded

Soak seeds and almonds overnight in water to cover, then drain before using. Using the metal S blade in the food processor, add the nuts, seeds, carrots, garlic, and onion. Remove from food processor and mix in the finely chopped parsley, red pepper, and celery. Grind the meat in the food processor and knead into the mix.

Blend the tomato and tomato paste with the oregano, basil, black pepper, and chili powder. Fold three-fourths of the tomato sauce into the mixture, leaving the remains to baste over the cooking loaf. Form the mix into a loaf and refrigerate for a few hours or freeze for one hour until ready to cook. Bake in oven at 300 degrees for one hour, basting with the tomato sauce at approximately 20 minutes and 40 minutes. Serve on a bed of shredded lettuce.

WILD RICE AND BROCCOLI
Serves 4–6

1 cup wild rice
1 cup brown rice
1 tablespoon garlic powder
1 tablespoon onion powder
1 tablespoon oregano flakes
2 large bunches broccoli, cut up
2 tablespoons olive oil

Use a very large pot to simmer the 2 cups of rice with 5 cups of water and the seasonings on a low heat for 30 minutes. Then add the pieces of broccoli on top of the rice, sprinkle the olive oil over the broccoli, and let simmer another 15 minutes, until the broccoli is soft. Toss and serve.

FRUIT DISHES/BREAKFAST FOODS
AND DESSERTS

....

ALMOND CAROB FUDGE
Serves 4

½ cup dates
¼ cup soy milk
1 cup raw almond butter
½ cup raw carob powder
½ cup shredded coconut
1 teaspoon vanilla extract

Chop dates and cover overnight with the soy milk to soften. Mash and mix all ingredients, including the soy milk soak, together and press in glass dish. Chill in refrigerator or freezer before cutting to serve.

APPLE PECAN PUDDING
Serves 3–6

6 peeled and cored apples, dried
2 cups soy milk
2 cups pecans
¼ teaspoon nutmeg
1 tablespoon cinnamon
5 medjool dates
2 cups organic sun-dried apples

Soak dried apples in soy milk overnight. Blend with remaining ingredients in the morning and place in muffin pan or a few small ceramic ovenware bowls. Cook at 200 degrees for 20 minutes. Cool in refrigerator before serving.

APPLE WALNUT SURPRISE
Serves 6

1 cup raisins or currents
½ cup water
8–10 apples, peeled and cored
½ cup finely chopped walnuts
4 heaping tablespoons ground flax seeds
1½ heaping tablespoons ground cinnamon

Soak raisins or currents in the water in a container with a closed top overnight in the refrigerator to soften. Poor off the water into a pot with a tight lid and add the peeled and cored apples. Let simmer over a low flame for 7 minutes. Pour the apples and the little liquid that remains off into a chopping bowl or hand chopper and dice up the softened apples into small pieces. Mix the apples, raisins, walnuts, flax seeds, and cinnamon in a bowl and mix well. Store in refrigerator to serve for meals and snacks.

BAKED APPLE WITH CASHEW RAISIN CREAM SAUCE
Serves 4

4 large apples
1 cup raw cashew nuts
1 cup soy milk
1 cup raisins
1 teaspoon cinnamon

Core apples and place on silver-foil-covered baking pan. Blend cashews, soy milk, and raisins to make cream sauce and chill. Sprinkle apples with cinnamon and bake at 200 for 20 minutes in oven. Move from baking dish to serving dish, pour chilled cream sauce on top, and serve.

BANANA NUT COOKIES
Yields 25 cookies

¼ cup pitted dates
¼ cup regular soy milk
1 cup walnuts
1 cup pecans
1 cup grated coconut
4 ripe bananas
2 teaspoons cinnamon

Cover dates in soy milk and soak overnight. Place the nuts and coconut in a food processor with the metal S blade and grind to a coarse meal. Add the bananas, dates (with the soaking soy milk), and cinnamon and mix to form the dough. Take the thick mixture out of the food processor and spoon onto a nonstick cookie sheet. Bake in the oven at a low heat (250 degrees) for 30 minutes.

BANANA/PINEAPPLE SORBET
Serves 2

1 frozen banana, sliced
1 small (4-ounce) can unsweetened pineapple or fresh pineapple

Whip the frozen banana with the pineapple and serve immediately.

BLUEBERRY AND FLAX YOGURT
Serves 1

2 cups fresh or frozen blueberries
½ cup regular soy milk
1 tablespoon ground flax seeds
3 medjool or 6 Deglet Noor dates

Blend until smooth. Chill and serve. Great for school lunches, too.

CANTALOUPE SLUSH
Serves 2–4

1 cantaloupe
2 cups ice
6–8 dates

Blend the ingredients together in a Vita-Mix or other high-powered blender or food processor until smooth. The same drink can be made with peaches or nectarines. Date sugar can be used instead of the dates.

CAROB-AVOCADO CREAM PIE
Serves 4

Crust:
¼ cup unsweetened shredded coconut
½ cup crushed raw macadamia nuts
2 date-coconut rolls or 4 medjool dates

Mash coconut, macadamia, and dates together and keep kneading until well mixed. Press the mixture into a glass pie pan.

Creamy Filling:

2 tablespoons raw carob powder

12 raw cashews

1 avocado

3 medjool or 8 regular-size dates

Blend the carob, cashews, avocado, and dates together in a Vita-Mix or food processor until creamy and smooth. Spoon filling over crust and chill by freezing for one hour before serving.

DATE NUT POP'EMS

(3–6 Servings)

1 cup of ground nuts: cashews, walnuts, sunflower seeds, and almonds (cashew butter can be substituted for the ground cashews)

2 date coconut rolls or 3 soft medjool dates

Grind the nuts and seeds in a high-powered blender or coffee grinder to make a fine nut flour. I often use the back of a wooden spoon to crush the walnuts into a paste. Knead the date roll or mashed medjool dates into the powdered/crushed nuts. Add the cashew butter if desired and continue to knead until an even consistency. Mold into bite-size balls so toddlers can use as finger food. You can grind a large amount of the nuts at one time and store in the freezer for later use.

FLAX/OATMEAL BARS
Serves 4

½ cup dried apples
½ cup raisins
½ cup dates
1½ cups vanilla soy milk
1 cup rolled oats or oat flakes
3 tablespoons ground flax seeds
1 tablespoon raw cashew butter or peanut butter

Soak apples, raisins, and dates in half the soy milk in refrigerator overnight. Mix oats and ground flax seeds together and soak likewise with the other half of the soy milk in refrigerator overnight. In the morning, blend the dried fruit mix in a blender or food processor with the nut butter. Mix the blended fruit with the oat/flax seed mixture and roll into logs or spread on baking tray. Cook in oven on low heat (200 degrees) for 30 minutes to dehydrate.

FUHRMAN FUDGSICLES
Serves 6–8

2 ripe bananas
1 cup cashew nuts
2 tablespoons carob powder
½ teaspoon vanilla extract

Blend ingredients together in blender or food processor. Spoon out into Tupperware ice pop tray and freeze. Rinse outside of popsicle tray with hot water to pull the pops out of the tray easily.

PEACH SORBET
Serves 2–3

1 pound frozen peaches
¼ cup soy milk
4 dates

Blend ingredients until silky smooth in food processor, Vita-Mix, or other good blender.

RICE PUDDING WITH BANANA/APRICOT SAUCE
Serves 4

1 cup dried apricots
1 cup raisins
2 cups soy milk
3 egg whites
10 dates
1 tablespoon cinnamon
1 teaspoon vanilla
4 cups cooked brown rice
1 banana

Soak apricots and raisins in the soy milk, each in its own separate closed container, in the refrigerator overnight. The next day pour off the soy milk from the raisins into the blender with the egg whites, dates, cinnamon, and vanilla. Mix with the rice and raisins and place in shallow baking pan. Bake at 250 degrees for 30 minutes. Chill before serving.

Blend one banana with the soaked apricots and soy milk and pour over chilled bowls of rice pudding.

SOY MILK FRUIT SMOOTHIES
Serves 2

1 banana
2 cups soy milk
2–4 dates
8–16 ounces frozen fruit

Use a blender or food processor to make these tasty fruit drinks. Use 1 banana, 2 cups soy milk, and a few dates, plus an assortment of fresh and frozen fruit such as cherries, blueberries, strawberries, mangos, and peaches, to make a great fun drink.

TUTTIE FRUITIE PITA SANDWICH
Serves 3

1 cup dried mango
1 cup soy milk
1 banana
1 avocado
¼ cup almonds
3 whole-grain pita pockets, cut in half

Soak dried mango in soy milk overnight. Drain off soy milk and blend with banana, avocado, and almonds. Thicken the mixture by letting it dehydrate in a low-heat 200-degree oven for 30 minutes. You can leave the oven door open a crack to keep the temperature a little lower. Spread mixture into the inside of one side of each pita and lay the soaked dried mango over the other side. Lightly toast the pita and wrap with silver foil for a great school lunch treat.

VANILLA-CAROB FUDGE
Serves 4

1½ cups almonds
½ cup raw tahini
2 tablespoons honey
1 teaspoon vanilla
1 tablespoon raw carob powder

Process almonds in food processor and then add tahini, honey, and vanilla. Process until well mixed. Press half the mixture in a square baking dish and then add the carob powder to the rest of the mix and process. Drop spoonfuls of the carob mixture on top of the plain mixture and then carefully spread it over the top until evenly distributed. Refrigerate for at least an hour and enjoy!

WHIPPED BANANA FREEZE
Serves 2–3

2 peeled frozen bananas (one per person)
frozen strawberries or blueberries (optional)
¼ cup unsweetened soy milk
½ teaspoon vanilla
1 tablespoon of ground flax seed per person
1 tablespoon of crushed walnuts per person

Cut up the frozen fruit into small pieces. Put the soy milk, bananas, and vanilla into a Vita-Mix, blender, or food processor and blend until smooth. Sprinkle ground flax or crushed walnuts on top.

WHIPPED CREAM AND STRAWBERRIES
Serves 4–6

1⅓ cups macadamia nuts
1 cup soy milk
⅔ cup dates

Blend nuts, soy milk, and dates to make the best-tasting whipped cream. Eat with fresh or frozen strawberries (defrosted).

A variation on this theme is to soak dried mangoes in the soy milk overnight and use fewer dates.

TEN DAYS OF SUGGESTED MENUS

Keep in mind that in the real world, leftovers are used in the next day or two, so the ten days of meal plans here could take almost a month to go through. These are mostly vegetarian meal plans, but there are three dishes chosen out of the eighty below (comprising 30 meals) that are made with animal products. Those same recipes can be made without the animal products for vegetarians. If you decide to include animal products in your family diet, utilize them in the manner below, only about two to three times a week and as part of a vegetable dish; either way, you are following a plant-based diet.

* = From recipe section on pages 178–212.

DAY 1

Breakfast: Assorted fresh fruits
Cinnamon Apple Oatmeal
Lunch: Tomato Tornado Soup*
Apricot Brown Rice*
Fresh fruit

Dinner: Spinach Salad with Orange/Cashew Dressing*
Squash Fantasia*
Cantaloupe Slush*

DAY 2

Breakfast: Fresh-squeezed orange juice
Whole-grain bread spread with raw almond butter and
a mashed date roll
Lunch: Green salad with balsamic vinaigrette dressing
Pita pocket stuffed with shredded carrots, brown rice,
and sesame tahini
Fresh fruit
Dinner: Split Pea and Tofu Dog Soup*
String Beans and Almond Dust*
Healthy Potato Fries*
Melon balls

DAY 3

Breakfast: Cup of strawberries (fresh or frozen)
Apple Walnut Surprise*
Lunch: Pita pocket stuffed with lettuce, avocado, and Hot
Russian Dressing*
Fruit compote: dried apricots, frozen peaches, oats
soaked the night before in soy or skim milk
Dinner: Patriotic Salad*
Steamed asparagus
Veggie Meat Loaf*
Peach Sorbet*

DAY 4

Breakfast: Assorted fresh fruits
British Baked Tofu*
Lunch: Cabbage Raisin Soup*
Apples, raw brazil nuts, and raw pistachio nuts
Dinner: Spinach salad with hard-boiled egg whites, shredded apples, crushed walnuts, cinnamon, and toasted sesame seeds
Corn on the cob
Baked beans or mild vegetarian chili (canned from the health food store) with shredded lettuce
Watermelon

DAY 5

Breakfast: Cup of blueberries (fresh or frozen)
Baked Apple with Cashew Raisin Cream Sauce*
Lunch: Peachy Leek Soup*
Apple slices coated with cashew butter
Carrot sticks and cherry tomatoes with hummus dip
Dinner: Green Banana Power Blended Salad*
Chocolate Lentils*
Sweet potatoes
Banana Nut Cookies*

DAY 6

Breakfast: Fresh-squeezed orange juice
Cinnamon apple oatmeal
Lunch: Whole-wheat bread, lettuce, tomatoes, Hot Russian Dressing,* and sliced turkey breast, or use sliced avocado instead of turkey
Grapes or cherries

Dinner:　　Pecan Maple Salad*

Steamed artichokes

Eggplant Sicilian*

Fresh or unsweetened canned pineapple

DAY 7

Breakfast: Cup of mixed frozen berries

Banana mashed with avocado

Lunch:　　Purple Potato Salad*

Carrot Cream Soup*

Fruit

Dinner:　　Romaine lettuce and tomato salad with olive oil

Tofu Pizza Slices*

California Creamed Kale*

Banana/Pineapple Sorbet*

DAY 8

Breakfast: Cantaloupe slush*

Oatmeal with cinnamon, walnuts, and raisins

Lunch:　　Raw veggies (cherry tomatoes, sliced peppers, carrots)

with Red-Hot Hummus*

Tuttie Fruitie Pita Sandwich*

Dinner:　　Fresh fruit and raw nuts

Raw celery, fennel (sweet anise), and red peppers

spread with cashew or almond butter or a dip made

with the leftover hummus mixed with baked eggplant

Rice Pudding with Banana/Apricot Sauce*

DAY 9

Breakfast: Whipped Banana Freeze*

Whole-grain bread, toasted, and avocado spread

Lunch: Broccoli with melted soy cheese on top

Blueberry and Flax Yogurt*

Dinner: Green salad with Orange Cashew Dressing*

Quinoa and Nut Loaf*

Steamed string beans

Carob-Avocado Cream Pie*

DAY 10

Breakfast: Soy milk fruit smoothie*

Lunch: Brown rice, kidney bean chili, shredded lettuce

Fresh fruit

Dinner: Carrot Cream Soup*

Peas and corn

Teriyaki Chicken Coleslaw*

Whipped Cream and Strawberries*

....

Final Word

The knowledge you have gained from reading this book can give you the power to shape your child's health destiny.

But this book was not written only to benefit your child. You, too, can retard the aging process; maintain a healthy weight; lower your blood pressure; prevent or reverse diabetes; protect yourself against heart disease, stroke, and the so-common mental decline seen with aging; and overall live a better quality, healthier and longer life.

I hope you will join me on this road to wellness and bring as many people along for the ride as possible. Too many people suffer and die needlessly, and I'm sure millions of people of all ages would adopt a healthier diet style if they learned the profound benefits they would receive and how delicious it can be.

Learning what is necessary to establish good health is a tremendous first step, but not the entire solution. The rest of the story is the art of being a thoughtful, understanding parent, bending when we need to bend and remaining firm when that is in the best interests of our child. There are no simple rules to follow. I am sure what you have learned here can help you to be better parents, but it won't always be easy. Society will place many obstacles in your path. There will be times when you will not be perfect, and neither will your child. However, as time goes on and you strive to live a healthier life, nutritious eating will become a habit and you will find it easier and easier.

Moving your family in a healthier direction is a process that requires time, effort, and the ability to learn from past mistakes. Don't get discouraged if you fall back and make mistakes; just never give up.

Now that you have read this book and gained an understanding of information dear to my heart, you have become a member of my community, too, a community of health-conscious people striving to live sanely in today's world. Please send me your stories, and let me know of your difficulties and your triumphs. I will be excited to hear from you.

I wish you and your children a wonderful life, full of laughter and enduring health.

Visit Dr. Fuhrman at www.DrFuhrman.com.

List of Abbreviations

Acta Cardiol	Acta Cardiologica
Acta Otolaryngo	Acta Oto-Laryngologica
Acta Paediatr Jpn	Acta Paediatrica Japonica
Aliment Pharmacol Ther	Aliment Pharmacology and Therapeutics
Altern Med Rev	Alternative Medicine Review
Am Acad Child Adolesc	American Academy of Children and Adolescence
Ambul Pediatr	Ambulatory Pediatrics
Am J Cardiol	American Journal of Cardiology
Am J Clin Nutr	American Journal of Clinical Nutrition
Am J Epidemiol	American Journal of Epidemiology
Am J Health Promot	American Journal of Health Promotion
Am J Hypertens	American Journal of Hypertension
Am J Kidney Ds	American Journal of Kidney Disease
Am J Med	American Journal of Medicine
Am J Physiol	American Journal of Physiology
Am J Psychiatry	American Journal of Psychiatry
Am J Publ Health	American Journal of Public Health
Ann Allergy Asthma Immunol	Annals of Allergy, Asthma, and Immunology
Ann Emerg Med	Annals of Emergency Medicine
Ann Intern Med	Annals of Internal Medicine
Ann Med	Annals of Medicine
Ann NY Acad Sci	Annals of the New York Academy of Sciences

Annu Rev Nutr	Annual Review of Nutrition
Appl Psychophysiol Biofeedback	Applied Psychophysiology and Biofeedback
Arch Intern Med	Archives of Internal Medicine
Arch Pediatr Adolesc Med	Archives of Pediatrics and Adolescent Medicine
Arch Latinoam Nutr	Archivos LatinoAmericanos De Nutricion
Arch Neurol	Archives of Neurology
Best Pract Res Clin Endocrinol	Best Practical Research in Clinical Endocrinology
Biomed Environ	Biomedical Environment
Breast Cancer Res Treat	Breast Cancer Research and Treatment
Br J BioMed Sci	British Journal of Biomedical Science
Br J Cancer	British Journal of Cancer
Br J Nutr	British Journal of Nutrition
Brit Med J	British Medical Journal
Calcif Tissue Int	Calcified Tissue International
Can J Gastroenterol	Canadian Journal of Gastroenterology
Can J Psychiatry	Canadian Journal of Psychiatry
Canad J Surg	Canadian Journal of Surgery
Cancer Causes Control	Cancer Causes and Control
Cancer Epidemiol Biomarkers Prev	Cancer Epidemiology Biomarkers and Prevention
Cancer J Clin	Cancer Journal for Clinicians
Cancer Res	Cancer Research
Clin Endocrinol Metab	Clinical Endocrinology and Metabolism
Clin Exp Allergy	Clinical and Experimental Allergy
Clin Microbiol Rev	Clinical Microbiology Reviews
Cochrane Database Syst Rev	Cochrane Database of Systemic Review
Curr Allergy Asthma Rep	Current Allergy and Asthma Report
Curr Atheroscler Rep	Current Atherosclerosis Report
Curr Opin Lipidol	Current Opinion in Lipidology
Curr Probl Pediatr	Current Problems in Pediatrics
Eur J Cancer	European Journal of Cancer Prevention
Eur J Clin Nutr	European Journal of Clinical Nutrition
Eur Respir J	European Respiratory Journal
Food Addit Contam	Food Additives and Contaminants
Food Chem Toxicol	Food and Chemical Toxicology
Intl J Eating Disord	International Journal of Eating Disorders
Int J Cancer	International Journal of Cancer
Intl J Food Sci Nutr	International Journal of Food Science and Nutrition
Intl J Obes	International Journal of Obesity

Int J Obes Relat Metab Disord	International Journal of Obesity and Related Metabolic Disorders
Int J Pediatr Otorhinolaryngol	International Journal of Pediatric Otorhinolaryngology
Int J Toxicol	International Journal of Toxicology
J Allergy Clin Immunol	Journal of Allergy and Clinical Immunology
J Altern Complement Med	Journal of Alternative and Complementary Medicine
J Am Diet Assoc	Journal of the American Dietetic Association
J Am Acad Child Adolesc Psychiatry	Journal of the American Academy of Child and Adolescent Psychiatry
J Am Board Fam Pract	Journal of the American Board of Family Practice
J Am Coll Nutr	Journal of the American College of Nutrition
J Am Dietetic Asso	Journal of the American Dietetic Association
J Am Med Assoc	Journal of the American Medical Association
J Clin Microbiol	Journal of Clinical Microbiology
J Clin Oncol	Journal of Clinical Oncology
J Epidemiol Community Health	Journal of Epidemiology and Community Health
J Fam Pract	Journal of Family Practice
J Food Prot	Journal of Food Protection
J Gen Intern Med	Journal of General Internal Medicine
J Lipid Res	Journal of Lipid Research
J Med Microbiol	Journal of Medical Microbiology
J Natl Can Inst	Journal of the National Cancer Institute
J Nurs Res	Journal of Nursing Research
J Nutr	Journal of Nutrition
J Nutr Health Aging	Journal of Nutrition, Health and Aging
J Nutr Sci Vitaminol	Journal of Nutritional Science and Vitaminology
J Pediatr	Journal of Pediatrics
J Paediatr Child Health	Journal of Paediatrics and Child Health
J Toxicol Clin Toxicol	Journal of Toxicology Clinical Toxicology
J Urol	Journal of Urology
Life Sci	Life Sciences
Med Hypotheses	Medical Hypotheses
Med J Aust	Medical Journal of Australia

Med Sci Sports & Exerc	Medicine and Science in Sports and Exercise
Metab	Metabolism
Mutat Res	Mutation Research
N Eng J Med	New England Journal of Medicine
Nutr Cancer	Nutrition and Cancer
Nutr Health	Nutrition and Health
Nutr Neurosci	Nutritional Neurosciences
Nutr Rep Intl	Nutrition Reports International
Nutr Res	Nutritional Research
Nutr Rev	Nutrition Reviews
Pediatr Nephrol	Pediatric Nephrology
Pharmacol Res	Pharmacological Research
Physiol Res	Physiological Research
Presse Med	Presse Medicale
Prev Med	Preventive Medicine
Prog Neuropsychopharmacol Biol Psychiatry	Progress in Neuro-Psychopharmacology and Biological Psychiatry
Prostaglandins Leukot Essent	Prostaglandins Leukotrienes and Essential Fatty Acids
Rev Food Sci Nutr	Review of Food Science and Nutrition
Respir Med	Respiratory Medicine
Saudi Med J	Saudi Medical Journal
Scand J Immunol	Scandinavian Journal of Immunology
Toxicol Lett	Toxicology Letters
Trends Mol Med	Trends in Molecular Medicine
Ugeskr Laeger	Ugeskrift for Laeger

···········

Notes

INTRODUCTION: WE ARE MOLDED BY OUR CHILDHOOD

1. Fox MK, Pac S, Devaney B, Jankowski L. Feeding infants and toddlers study: What foods are infants and toddlers eating? *J Am Diet Assoc* 2004;104(1 Suppl):s22–s30.

2. Vincent SD, Pangrazi RP, Raustorp LM, et al. Activity levels and body mass index of children in the United States, Sweden and Australia. *Med Sci Sports & Exerc* 2003;35(8);1367–1373.

1. UNDERSTANDING SUPERIOR NUTRITION

1. Kim Y. Folate and cancer-prevention: a new medical application of folate beyond hyperhomocysteinemia and neural tube defects. *Nutr Rev* 1999;57(10):314–321. Lucock M, Daskalakis I. New perspectives on folate status: a differential role for the vitamin in cardiovascular diseases, birth defects and other conditions. *Br J Biomed Sci* 2000:57(3):254–260.

2. Jensen CD, Block G, Buffler P, et al. Maternal dietary factors in childhood acute lymphoblastic leukemia. *Cancer Causes Control* 2004;15(6):559–570.

3. Ames BN. Micronutrients prevent cancer and delay aging. *Toxicol Lett* Dec 28, 1998;102–103:5–18. Ames BN, DNA damage from micronutrient deficiencies is likely to be a major cause of cancer. *Mutat Res* 2001:475(1–2):7–20.

4. Burkitt, DP, Walker ARP, Painter NS. Dietary fiber and disease. *J Am Med Assoc* 1974;229:1068–1074.

5. Kromhout D. Serum cholesterol in cross-cultural perspective. The Seven Countries Study. *Act Cardiol* 1999;54(3):155–158.

6. Lichtenstein AH, Kennedy E, Barrier P, et al. Dietary fat consumption and health. *Nutr Rev* 1998;56 (5 pt2):S3–S28.

7. Kromhout D, Menotti A, Bloemberg B, et al. Dietary saturated and trans fatty

acids and cholesterol and 25-year mortality form coronary heart disease; the Seven Countries Study. *Prev Med* 1995;24(3):308–315. Oomen CM, Ocke MC, Feskens EJ, et al. Association between trans fatty acid intake and 10-year risk of coronary heart disease in the Zutphen Elderly study: a prospective population-based study. *Lancet* 2001;357(9258):746–751. Lemaitre RN, King IB, Raghunathan TE, et al. Cell membrane trans-fatty acids and the risk of primary cardiac arrest. *Circulation* 2002;105(6):697–701. Kromhout D. Diet and cardiovascular diseases. *J Nutr Health Aging* 2001;5(3):144–149.

8. Hu FB, Manson JE, Willett WC. Types of dietary fat and risk of coronary heart disease: a critical review. *J Am Coll Nutr* 2001;20(1):5–19.

9. Lichtenstein AH, Van Horn L. Very low fat diets. *Circulation* 1998;98(9):935–939.

10. Slattery ML, Benson J, Ma KN, et al. Trans-fatty acids and colon cancer. *Nutr Cancer* 2001;39(2):170–175. Kohlmeier L, Simonsen N, Van't Veer P, et al. Adipose tissue trans fatty acids and breast cancer in the European Community multicenter study on antioxidants, myocardial infarction and breast cancer. *Cancer Epidemiol Biomarkers Prev* 1997;6(9):705–710.

11. Lichtenstein AH. Trans Fatty acids and cardiovascular disease risk. *Curr Opin Lipidol* 2000;11(1):37–42.

12. *Composition of Foods—Raw-Processed-Prepared, Agriculture Handbook 8.* Series and Supplements. United States Department of Agriculture, Human Nutrition Information Service, Minnesota Nutrition Data System (NDS) software, developed by the Nutrition Coordinating Center, University of Minnesota, Minneapolis, MN. Food Database version 5A, Nutrient Database version 20, USDA Nutrient Database for Standard Reference. Release 14 at www.nal.usda.gov.fnic.

13. Exler J, Lerner L, Smith J. Fat and Fatty Acid Content of Selected Foods Containing Trans-Fatty Acids. Special Purpose Table No. 1. U.S. Department of Agriculture. Beltsville Human Nutrition Research Center. Nutrient Data Laboratory. www.nal.usda.gov/fnic.foodcomp.

14. Konings EJ, Baars AJ, van Klaveren JD, et al. Acrylamide exposure from foods of the Dutch population and an assessment of the consequent risks. *Food Chem Toxicol* 2003;41(11):1569–1579.

15. Albert CM, Gaziano JM, Willett WC, Manson JE. Nut consumption and decreased risk of sudden cardiac death in the Physicians' Health Study. *Arch Intern Med* 2002;162(12):1382–1387.

16. Sabate J. Nut consumption, vegetarian diets, ischemic heart disease risk, and all-cause mortality; evidence from epidemiologic studies. *Am J Clin Nutr* 1999;70(3 Suppl):500S–503S. Hu FB, Stampfer MJ. Nut consumption and risk of coronary heart disease: a review of epidemiologic evidence. *Curr Atheroscler Rep* 1999;1(3):204–209.

17. McKeever TM, Lewis SA, Smith C, et al. Early exposure to infections and antibiotics and the incidence of allergic disease: a birth cohort study with the West Midlands General Practice Research Database. *J Allergy Clin Immunol* 2002;109(1):43–50. Holen E, Elsayed S. Why does the prevalence of allergy increase more in industrialized countries than in developing countries? *Tidsskr Nor Laegeforen* (Norway) 1999;119(21):3176–3177.

18. Mortensen EL; Michaelsen KF; Sanders SA; Reinisch JM. The association between duration of breast-feeding and adult intelligence. *JAMA* 2002;287(18):2365–2371.

19. Ramakrishna T. Vitamins and brain development. *Physiol Res* 1999;48(3):175–187. Brown JL, Sherman LP. Policy implications of new scientific knowledge. *J Nutr* 1995;125(8S):2281S–2284S. Schoenthaler SJ, Bier ID, Young K, et al. The effect of vitamin-mineral supplementation on the intelligence of American schoolchildren: a randomized double-blind placebo-controlled trial. *J Altern Complement Med* 2000;6(1):19–29.

20. Leiva PB, Inzunza BN, Perez TH, et al. The impact of malnutrition on brain development, intelligence and school work performance. *Arch Latinoam Nutr* 2001;1(1):64–71.

21. Haag M. Essential fatty acids and the brain. *Can J Psychiatry* 2003;48(3):195–203.

22. Bowman S, Gortmaker S, Ebbeling C, et al. Effects of fast-food consumption on energy intake and diet quality among children in a national household survey. *Pediatrics* 2004;113(1):112–118.

23. Saelens BE, Ernst MM, Epstein LH. Maternal child feeding practices and obesity: a discordant sibling analysis. *Int J Eat Disord* 2000;27(4):459–463.

24. French SA, Lin BH, Guthrie JF. National trends in soft drink consumption among children and adolescents age 6 to 17 years: prevalence, amounts, and sources, 1977/1978 to 1994/1998. *J Am Diet Assoc* 2003;103(10):1326–1331.

25. Muntner P, He J, Cutler JA, et al. Trends in blood pressure among children and adolescents. *JAMA* 2004;291:2107–2113.

26. Tsugane S, Sasazuki S, Kobayashi M, Sasaki S. Salt and salted food intake and subsequent risk of gastric cancer among middle-aged Japanese men and women. *Br J Cancer* 2004;90(1):128–134. Ngoan LT, Mizoue T, Fujino Y, et al. Dietary factors and stomach cancer mortality. *Br J Cancer* 2002;87(1):37–42. Nozaki K, Tsukamoto T, Tatematsu M. Effect of high salt diet and Helicobacter pylori infection of gastric carcinogenesis. *Nippon Rinsho* 2003;61(1):36–40.

27. Geleijnse JM, Grobbee DE. High salt intake early in life: does it increases the risk of hypertension? *J Hypertens* 2002;20(11):2121–2124. Holiday MA. Is blood pressure in later life affected by events in infancy? *Pediatr Nephrol* 1995;9(5):663–666.

28. Langford HG, Watson RL. Close correlation between blood pressure and sodium excretion in hypertensives-to-be, abstracted. *Circulation* 1982;66(suppl 11):11–105.

29. Freis Ed. Salt, volume and the prevention of hypertension. *Circulation* 1976;54:589.

30. Young VR, Pellett PL. Plant proteins in relation to human protein and amino acid nutrition. *Am J Clin Nutr* 1994;59(suppl 5):1203S–1212S.

31. Jenkins DJ, Kendall CW, Popovich, et al. Effects of a very-high-fiber vegetable fruit and nut diet on serum lipids and colonic function. *Metabolism* 2001;50(4);494–503.

32. Rose W. The amino acid requirements of adult man. *Nutritional Abstracts and Reviews* 1957;27:631.

33. Hardage M. Nutritional studies of vegetarians. *Journal of the American Dietetic Association* 1966;48:25.

34. Barzel US, Massey LK. Excess dietary protein can adversely affect bone. *J Nutr*

1998;128(6):1051–1053. Itoh R, Suyama Y. Sodium excretion in relation to calcium and hydroxyproline excretion in healthy Japanese population. *Am J Clin Nutr* 1996;63(5): 735–740.

35. New SA, Robins SP, Campbell MK, et al. Dietary influences on bone mass and bone metabolism: further evidence of a positive link between fruit and vegetable consumption and bone health? *Am J Clin Nutr* 2000;71(1):142–151.

2. PREVENTING AND TREATING CHILDHOOD ILLNESSES NUTRITIONALLY

1. Taylor JA, Novack AH, Almquist JR, Rogers JE. Efficacy of cough suppressants in children. *J Pediatr* 1993 122;(5 Pt 1):799–802.

2. Shatin D; Drinkard CR. Ambulatory use of psychotropics by employer-insured children and adolescents in a national managed care organization. *Ambul Pediatr* 2002;2(2):111–119.

3. McCormick LH. ADHD treatment and academic performance: A case series. *J Family Practice* 2003;52(8):620–624. Cantwell DP, Baker L. Attention deficit disorder with and without hyperactivity; a review and comparison of matched groups. *J Am Acad Child Adolesc Psychiatry* 1992;31:432–438. Barkley RA, DuPaul GJ, McMurray MB. Attention deficit disorder with and without hyperactivity: clinical response to three dose levels of methylphenidate. *Pediatrics* 1991;87:519–531. Safer DJ. Major treatment consideration for attention hyperactivity disorder. *Curr Probl Pediatr* 1995;25:137–143.

4. Dunnick JK, Hailey JR. Experimental studies on the long-term effects of methylphenidate hydrochloride. *Toxicology* 1995;103(2):77–84.

5. Boris M, Mandel FS. Foods and additives are common causes of the attention deficit hyperactive disorder in children. *Ann Allergy* 1994 May;72(5):462–468. Krummel DA, Seligson FH, Guthria HA. Hyperactivity: is candy causal? *Rit Rev Food Sci Nutr* 1996;36:31–47. Dulcan M. Practice parameters for the assessment and treatment of children, adolescents, and adults with attention-deficit/hyperactivity disorder. *AJ Am Acad Child Adolesc Psychiatry* 1997;36:85S–121S.

6. Breakey J. The role of diet and behaviour in childhood. *J Paediatr Child Health* 1997;33(3):190–194. Schnoll R, Burshteyn D, Cea-Aravena J. Nutrition in the treatment of attention-deficit hyperactivity disorder: a neglected but important aspect. *Appl Psychophysiol Biofeedback* 2003;28(1):63–75. Richardso AJ; Puri BK. A randomized double-blind, placebo-controlled study of the effects of supplementation with highly unsaturated fatty acids on ADHD-related symptoms in children with specific learning difficulties. *Prog Neuropsychopharmacol Biol Psychiatry* 2002;26(2):233–239. Kidd PM. Attention deficit/hyperactivity disorder (ADHD) in children: rationale for its integrative management. *Altern Med Rev* 2000;5(5):402–428.

7. Christakis DA, Zimmerman FJ, Di Giuseppe DL, et al. Early television exposure and subsequent attentional problems in children. *Pediatrics* 2004, 113(4):708–713.

8. Haag M. Essential fatty acids and the brain *Can J Psychiatry* 2003;48(3):195–203.

9. Mortensen EL; Michaelsen KF; Sanders SA; Reinisch JM. The association between duration of breast-feeding and adult intelligence. *JAMA* 2002;287(18):2365–2371.

10. Helland IB, Smith L, Saarem K, et al. Maternal supplementation with very-long-chain n-3 fatty acids during pregnancy and lactation augments children's IQ at 4 years of age. *Pediatrics* 2003;111(1):e39–40.

11. Horrocks LA, Yeo YK. Health benefits of docosahexaenoic acid (DHA). *Pharmacol Res* 1999;40(3):211–225.

12. Turner N, Else PL, Hulbert AJ. Docosahexaenoic acid (DHA) content of membranes determines molecular activity of the sodium pump: implication for disease states and metabolism. *Naturwissenschaften* 2003;90(11):521–523. Saugstad LF. Human nature is unique in the mismatch between the usual diet and the need for "food for the brain" (marine fat, DHA). Adding marine fat is beneficial in schizophrenia and manic-depressive psychosis. This underlines [that] brain dysfunction in these neurological disorders is associated with deficient intake of marine fat (DHA). *Nutr Health* 2002;16(1):41–44.

13. Horrocks LA, Yeo YK. Health benefits of docosahexaenoic acid (DHA). *Pharmacol Res* 1999 Sep;40(3):211–225. Haag M Essential fatty acids and the brain. *Can J Psychiatry* 2003;48(3):195–203. Richardson AJ, Puri BK. The potential role of fatty acids in attention-deficit/hyperactivity disorder. *Prostaglandins Leukot Essent Fatty Acids* 2000;63(1–2):79–87. Richardso AJ, Puri BK. A randomized double-blind, placebo-controlled study of the effects of supplementation with highly unsaturated fatty acids on ADHD-related symptoms in children with specific learning difficulties. *Prog Neuropsychopharmacol Biol Psychiatry* 2002;26(2):233–239.

14. Stevens, L, et al. Essential fatty acid metabolism in boys with attention-deficit hyperactivity disorder. *Am J Clin Nutr* 1995;62(4):761–768.

15. Steinman MA, Gonzales R, Linder JA, Landefeld CS. Changing use of antibiotics in community-based outpatient practice, 1991–1999. *Ann Intern Med* 2003;138(7):525–533.

16. Linder JA, Singer DE. Desire for antibiotics and antibiotic prescribing for adults with upper respiratory tract infections. *J Gen Intern Med* 2003;18(10):795–801. Nash DR, Harman J, Wald ER, Kelleher KJ. Antibiotic prescribing by primary care physicians for children with upper respiratory tract infections. *Arch Pediatr Adolesc Med* 2002;156(11):1114–1119.

17. Stone S, Gonzales R, Maselli J, Lowenstein SR. Antibiotic prescribing for patients with colds, upper respiratory tract infections, and bronchitis: A national study of hospital-based emergency departments. *Ann Emerg Med* 2000;36(4):320–327.

18. DiFrancesco E. Stop treating colds with antibiotics. *Infectious Disease News Aug* 1992;12. Orr PH, Scherer KS, Macdonald A, Moffatt MEK. Randomized placebo-controlled trials of antibiotics for acute bronchitis: A critical review of the literature. *J Fam Pract* 1993;36:507–512.

19. Betran AP, de Onis M, Lauer JA, Villar J. Ecological study of effect of breast-feeding on infant mortality in Latin America. *BMJ* 2001;323(7308):303–306. Abdulmoneim I, Al-Ghamdi SA. Relationship between breast-feeding duration and acute respiratory infection in infants. *Saudi Med J* 2001;22(4):347–350.

20. Pitkaranta A, Virolainen A, Jero J, et al. Detection of rhinovirus, respiratory syncytial virus, and coronavirus infections in acute otitis media by reverse transcriptase

polymerase chain reaction. *Pediatrics* 1998;102(2 Pt 1):291–295. Heikkinen T, Thint M, Chonmaitree T. Prevalence of various respiratory viruses in the middle ear during acute otitis media. *N Engl J Med* 1999;340(4):260–264. Heikkinen T, Chonmaitree T. Importance of respiratory viruses in acute otitis media. *Clin Microbiol Rev* 2003;16(2):230–241.

21. Tucker ME. When to use antibiotics—and when to resist. *Family Practice News* Dec 15, 1997; 27.

22. Heikkinen T, Chonmaitree T. Importance of respiratory viruses in acute otitis media. *Clin Microbiol Rev* 2003;16(2):230–241. Heikkinen T, Chonmaitree T. Increasing importance of viruses in acute otitis media. *Ann Med* 2000;32(3):157–163. Heikkinen T, Thint M, Chonmaitree T. Prevalence of various respiratory viruses in the middle ear during acute otitis media. *N Engl J Med* 1999;340(4):260–264. Pitkaranta A, Virolainen A, Jero J, et al. Detection of rhinovirus, respiratory syncytial virus, and coronavirus infections in acute otitis media by reverse transcriptase polymerase chain reaction. *Pediatrics* 1998;102(2 Pt 1):291–295.

23. Bollag U, Bollag-Albrecht E. Recommendations derived from practice audit for the treatment of acute otitis media. *Lancet* 1991;338(8759):96–99. Linder TE, Briner HR, Bischoff T. Prevention of acute mastoiditis: fact of fiction? *Int J Pediatr Otorhinolaryngol* 2000;56(2):129–134.

24. Glasziou PP, Del Mar CB, Hayem M, Sanders SL. Antibiotics for acute otitis media in children. *Cochrane Dantbase Syst Rev* 2000;(4):CD000219.

25. Froom J, Cupepper L, Green LA, et al. A cross-national study of acute otitis media; risk factors, severity, and treatment at initial visit. Report from the International Primary Care Network (IPCN) and the Ambulatory Sentinel Practice network (ASPN). *J Am Board Fam Pract* 2001;14(6):406–417.

26. Damoiseaux RA, van Balen FA, Hoes AW, et al. Primary care based randomized, double blind trial of amoxicillin versus placebo for acute otitis media in children aged under 2 years. *BMJ* 2000;320(7231):350–354.

27. McKeever TM, Lewis SA, Smith C, et al. Early exposure to infections and antibiotics and the incidence of allergic disease: a birth cohort study with the West Midlands General Practice Research Database. *J Allergy Clin Immunol* 2002;109(1):43–50. Wickens K, Pearce N, Crane J, Beasley R. Antibiotic use in early childhood and the development of asthma. *Clin Exp Allergy* 1999;29(6):766–771. Droste JH, Wieringa MH, Weyler JJ, et al. Does the use of antibiotics in early childhood increase the risk of asthma and allergic disease? *Clin Exp Allergy* 2000;30(11):1547–1553. Nelen VJ, Vermeire PA, Van Bever HP. Puzzling associations between childhood infections and the later occurrence of asthma and atopy. *Ann Med* 2000;32(6):397–400.

28. Eldeirawi K, Persky VW. History of ear infections and prevalence of asthma in a national sample of children aged 2 to 11 years: The Third National Health and Nutrition Examination Survey, 1988 to 1994. *Chest* 2004;125:1685–1692.

29. Card T, Logan RFA, Rodrigues LC, Wheeler JG. Antibiotic use and the development of Crohn's disease. *Gut* 2004;53:246–250.

30. Velicer CM, Heckbert SR, Lampe JW, et al. Antibiotic use in relation to the risk of breast cancer. *JAMA* 2004;291(7):827–835.

31. Iwata S, Akita H. Adverse effects of antibiotics. *Acta Paediatr Jpn* 1997 Feb;39(1): 143–154.

32. ATS 99th International Conference Mini-Symposium: Abstract Page A831. Risk Factors for the development of asthma in childhood (Hygiene Hypothesis)—Early life risk factors for asthma: findings from the Children's health Study. Presented May 21 2003.

33. Mellis CM. Is asthma prevention possible with dietary manipulation? *Med J Aust* 2002;177 Suppl:S78–S80.

34. Ushiyama Y, Matsumoto K, Shinohara M, et al. Nutrition during pregnancy may be associated with allergic disease in infants. *J Nutr Sci Vitaminol (Tokyo)* 2002;48(5):345–351.

35. Huang SL, Lin KC, Pan WH. Dietary factors associated with physician-diagnosed asthma and allergic rhinitis in teenagers: analysis of the first Nutrition and Health Survey in Taiwan. *Clin Exp Allergy* 2001;31(2):259–264. Huang SL, Pan Wh. Dietary fats and asthma in teenagers: analysis of the first Nutrition and Health Survey in Taiwan. *Clin Exp Allergy* 2001;31(12):1875–1880.

36. Hijazi N, Abalkham B, Seaton A. Diet and childhood asthma in a society in transition: a study in urban and rural Saudi Arabia. *Thorax* 2000;55(9):775–779. Denny SI, Thompson RL, Margetts BM. Dietary factors in the pathogenesis of asthma and chronic obstructive pulmonary disease. *Curr Allergy Asthma Rep* 2003;3(2):130–136.

37. Farchi S, Forastiere F, Agabiti N, et al. Dietary factors associated with wheezing and allergic rhinitis in children. *Eur Respir J* 2003;22(5):772–780.

38. Baker JC, Ayres JG. Diet and asthma. *Resp Med* 2000;94(10):925–934.

39. Host A. Frequency of cow's milk allergy in childhood. *Ann Allergy Asthma Immunol* 2002;89(6 Suppl. 1):33–37.

40. Dahl-Jorgensen K, Joner G, Hanssen KF. Relationship between cow's milk consumption and incidence of IDDM in childhood. *Diabetes Care* 1991;14(11):1081–1083.

41. Savilahti E, Saukkonen TT, Virtala ET, et al. Increased levels of cow's milk and beta-lactoglobulin antibodies in young children with newly diagnosed IDDM. The Childhood Diabetes in Finland Study Group. *Diabetes Care* 1993;16(7):984–989. Vaarala O, Paronen J, Otonkoski T, Akerblom HK. Cow milk feeding induces antibodies to insulin in children—a link between cow milk and insulin-dependent diabetes mellitus? *Scand J Immunol* 1998;47(2):131–135. Vahasalo P, Petays T, Knip M, et al. Relationship between antibodies to islet cell antigens, other autoantigens and cow's milk proteins in diabetic children and unaffected siblings at the clinical manifestation of IDDM. *Autoimmunity* 1996;23(3):165–174.

42. Kostraba JN, Cruickshanks KJ, Lawler-Heavner J, et al. Early exposure to cow's milk and solid foods in infancy, genetic predisposition, and risk of IDDM. *Diabetes* 1993;42(2):288–295.

43. Gerstein HC. Cow's milk exposure and type 1 diabetes mellitus. A critical overview of the clinical literature. *Diabetes Care* 1994;17(1):13–19. Hurley D. Studies confirm diabetes risk from cow's milk in infants. *Medical Tribune* 1995;Feb 2:11.

44. Collins AM, Xenogeneic antibodies and atopic disease. *Lancet* 1988 1(8588): 734–737.

45. Andiran F, Dayi S, Mete E. Cows milk consumption in constipation and anal fissure in infants and young children. *J Paediatr Child Health* 2003;39(5):329–331.

46. Iacono G, Cavataio F, Montalto G, et al. Intolerance of cow's milk and chronic constipation in children. *N Engl J Med* 1998;339(16):1100–1104.

47. Chamberlin W, Graham DY, Hulten K, et al. Review article: Mycobacterium avium subsp. Para tuberculosis as one cause of Crohn's disease. *Aliment Pharmacol Ther* 2001;15(3):337–346. El-Zaatari FA, Osato MS, Graham DY. Etiology of Crohn's disease: the role of Mycobacterium avium paratuberculosis. *Trends Mol Med* 2001;7(6):247–252.

48. Juntti H, Tikkanen S, Kokkenen J, et al. Cow's milk allergy is associated with recurrent otitis media during childhood. *Acta Otolaryngol* 1999;119(8):867–873.

49. Moss M, Freed D. The cow and the coronary: epidemiology, biochemistry and immunology. *Int J Cardiol* 2003;87(2–3):203–216. Strain JJ. Milk consumption, lactose and copper in the aetiology of ischaemic heart disease. *Med Hypothesis* 1988;25(2):99–101. Jacques H, Laurin D, Moorjani S, et al. Influence of diets containing cow's milk or soy protein beverage on plasma lipids in children with familial hypercholesterolemia. *J Am Coll Nutr* 1992;11(Suppl):69S–73S. Seely S. Possible connection between milk and coronary heart disease: the calcium hypothesis. *Med Hypotheses* 2000;54(5):701–703.

50. Malosse D, Perron H, Sasco A, Seigneurin JM. Correlation between milk and dairy product consumption and multiple sclerosis prevalence: a worldwide study. *Neuroepidemiology* 1992;11(4–6):304–312.

51. Gammaa D, Li XM, Wang J, et al. Incidence and mortality of testicular and prostatic cancers in relation to world dietary practices. *Int J Cancer* 2002 98(2):262–267.

52. Hermon-Taylor J, Bull TJ, Sheridan JM, et al. Causation of Crohn's disease by mycobacterium subspecies paratuberculosis. *Can J Gastroenterol* 2000;14(6):521–539. Harris JE, Lammerding AM. Crohn's disease and mycobacterium avium subsp. paratuberculosis: current issues. *J Food Prot* 2001;64(12):2103–2110. Chamberlin W, Graham DY, Hulten K, et al. Review article: Mycobacterium avium subsp. Paratuberculosis as one cause of Crohn's disease. *Aliment Pharmacol Ther* 2001;15(3):337–346. Hermon-Taylor J, Bull T. Crohn's disease caused by mycobacterium avium subspecies paratuberculosis: a public health tragedy whose resolution is long overdue. *J Med Microbiol* 2002;51(1):3–6. Lund BM, Gould GW, Rampling AM. Pasteurization of milk and the heat resistance of mycobacterium avium subsp. paratuberculosis: a critical review of the data. *Int J Food Microbiol* 2002;77(1–2):135–145. Detection and verification of mycobacterium avium subsp. paratuberculosis in fresh ileocolonic mucosal biopsy specimens from individuals with and without Crohn's Disease. *J Clin Microbiol* 2003;41(7): 2915–2923.

53. Taylor JH. Most of Crohn's disease and probably some irritable bowel syndrome is being caused by a bug called MAP (mycobacterium avium paratuberculosis). 104th general meeting of the American Society for Microbiology, May 20–27, 2004, New Orleans, La. (Session 127).

54. Dell S, To T. Breast-feeding and asthma in young children: findings from a population-based study. *Arch Pediatr Adolesc Med* 2001;155(11):1261–1265.

55. Ram FS, Ducharme FM, Scarlett J. Cow's milk protein avoidance and development of childhood wheeze in children with a family history of atopy. *Colchrane Database Syst* Rev 2002;(3):CD003795.

3. UNDERSTANDING THE CAUSES OF CANCER AND OTHER ILLNESSES

1. World Health Organization. *Prevention of cancer.* Geneva: World Health Organization,1964;Technical report series 276.

2. Jemal A, Tiwari RC, Murray T, et al. Cancer statistics, 2004. *CA Cancer J Clin* 2004;54:8–29.

3. Greenlee RT, Murray T, Bolden S, Wingo PA. Cancer statistics, 2000. *CA Cancer J Clin* 2000 Jan–Feb;50(1):7–33.

4. Doll R, Muir C, Waterhouse J. International Union Against Cancer (UICC). *Cancer Incidence in five continents.* Vol VI, Lyon 1997.

5. Ziegler RG, Hoover RN, Pike MC, et al. Migration patterns and breast cancer risk in Asian-American women. *J Natl Cancer Inst* 1993;85(22):1819–1827.

6. Boyd NF, Martin LJ, Noffel MM, et al. A meta-analysis of studies of dietary fat and breast cancer risk. *Br J Cancer* 1993;68:627–636. Steinmez KA, Potter JD, Vegetables, fruits and cancer prevention: a review. *J Am Diet Assoc* 1996;96(10):1067–39; La Vecchia C, Tavani A. Fruit and vegetable consumption and human cancer. *Eur J Cancer Prev* 1998;7(1):3–8.

7. Hursting SD, Thornquist M, Henderson. Types of dietary fat and the incidence of cancer at five sites. *Prev Med* 1990;19(3):242–53. Zhao LP, Kushi LH, Klein RD, et al. Quantitative review of studies of dietary fat and rat colon carcinoma. *Nutr Cancer* 1991;15(3–4):169–77. Fay MP, Freedman LS, Clifford CK, et al. Effect of different types and amounts of fat on the development of mammary tumors in rodents: a review. *Cancer Res* 1997;57(18):3979–88.

8. Brody J. Huge study of diet indicts fat and meat. *New York Times,* May 8, 2000.Science Times Section, p.1.

9. Campbell TC, Parpia B, Chen J. Diet, lifestyle, and the etiology of coronary artery disease: the Cornell China Study. *Am J Cardiol* 1998;82(10B):18–21T.

10. Littman AJ, Beresford SA, White E. The association of dietary fat and plant foods with endometrial cancer. *Cancer Causes Control* 2001;12(8):691–702. Hanash KA, Al-Othaimeen A, Kattan S, et al. Prostatic carcinoma: a nutritional disease? Conflicting data from the Kingdom of Saudi Arabia. *J Urol* 2000;164(5):1570–2. de la Taille A, Katz A, Vacherot F, et al. Cancer of the prostate: influence of nutritional factors. *Presse Med* 2001;30(11):554–6. Huncharek M, Kupelnick B. Dietary fat intake and risk of epithelial ovarian cancer: a meta-analysis of 6,689 subjects from 8 observational studies. *Nutr Cancer* 2001;40(2):87–91. Byrne C; Rockett H; Holmes MD Dietary fat, fat subtypes, and breast cancer risk: lack of an association among postmenopausal women with no history of benign breast disease. *Cancer Epidemiol Biomarkers Prev* 2002 Mar;11(3):261–5.

11. Willett WC, Hunter DJ, Stampfer MJ, et al. Dietary fat and fiber in relation to risk of breast cancer: An eight year follow-up. *JAMA* 1992;268(15):2037–44. Holmes MD,

Hunter DJ, Colditz GA, et al. Association of dietary intake of fat and fatty acids with risk of breast cancer. *JAMA* 1999;281(10):914–20. Holmes MD, Colditz GA, Hunter DJ, et al. Meat, fish, and egg intake and risk of breast cancer. 2003;104(2):221–227.

12. Dourson M, Charnley G, Scheuplein R. Differential sensitivity of children and adults to chemical toxicity. II. Risk and regulation. *Regul Toxicol Pharmacol* 2002;35(3): 448–467. Miller MD, Marty MA, Arcus A, et al. Differences between children and adults: implications for risk assessment at California EPA. *Int J Toxicol* 2002;21(5): 403–418.

13. Caygill C, Charlett A, Hill MJ. Relationship between the intake of high-fibre foods and energy and the risk of cancer of the large bowel and breast. *Euro J Cancer Prev* 1998;7(S2):S11–S17.

14. Engeland A, Tretli S, Bjorge T. Height, body mass index, and ovarian cancer: a follow-up of 1.1 million Norwegian women. *J Natl Cancer Inst* 2003;95:1244–1248.

15. Must A, Jacques PF, Dallal GF, et al. Long-term morbidity and mortality of over-weight adolescents: a follow-up of the Harvard Growth Study, 1922–1935. *N Eng J Med* 1992;327:1350–1355.

16. Barker DJ, Winter PD, Osmond C, et al. Weight gain in infancy and cancer of the ovary. *Lancet* 1995;345(8957):1087–1088.

17. Fairfield KM, Willett WC, Rosner BA, et al. Obesity, weight gain, and ovarian cancer. *Obstet Gynecol* 2002;100:288–296.

18. McPherson K, Steel CM, Dixon JM. ABC of Breast Diseases, Breast cancer—epidemiology, risk factors, and genetics. *BMJ* 2000;321:624–628. Pierce DA, Shimizu Y, Preston DL, et al. Studies of the mortality of atomic bomb survivors. Report 12, Part I. Cancer: 1950–1990 RERF Report No. 11-95. *Radiat Res* 1996;146:1–27.

19. Tsuji K, Harashima, E, Nakagawa Y, et al. Time-lag effect of dietary fiber and fat intake ratio on Japanese colon cancer mortality. *Biomed Environ* 1996;9(2–3):223–8.

20. Maynard M, Gunnell D, Emmett P, et al. Fruit, vegetable and antioxidants in childhood and risk of adult cancer: the Boyd Orr cohort. *J Epidemiol Community Health* 2003;57:218–225.

21. Erickson KL. Dietary pattern analysis: a different approach to analyzing an old problem, cancer of the esophagus and stomach. *Am J Clin Nutr* 2002;75(1):5–7. Satia-Abouta J, Galanko JA, Martin CF, et al. Food groups and colon cancer risk in African-Americans and Caucasians. *Int J Cancer* 2004;109(5):728–736.

22. Ward MH, Pan W, Cheng Y, et al. Dietary exposure to nitrate and nitrosamines and risk of nasopharyngeal carcinoma in Taiwan. *Int J Cancer* 2000;86:603–609.

23. Frankel S, Gunnell DJ, Peters TJ, et al. Childhood energy intake and adult mor-tality from cancer. *BMJ* 1998;316(7130):499–504.

24. Strauss RS, Pollack HA. Epidemic increase in childhood overweight, 1986–1998. *JAMA* 2001;286(22):2845–2848.

25. Okasha M. Gunnell D, Holly J, et al. Childhood growth and adult cancer. *Best Pract Res Clin Endocrinol Metab* 2002;16(2):225–41. Must A, Lipman RD, Childhood energy in-take and cancer mortality in adulthood. *Nutr Rev* 1999;57(1):21–4. Wang DY, De Stavola BL, Allen DS, et al. Breast cancer is positively associated with height. *Breast Cancer*

Res Treat 1997;43(2):123–8. Barker DJ, Winter PD, Osmond C, et al. Weight gain in infancy and cancer of the ovary. *Lancet* 1995;345(8957):1087–8. Albanes D, Jones DY, Schatzkin A, et al. Adult stature and risk of cancer. *Cancer Res* 1988;48:1658–62. Chute CG, Willett WC, Colditz GA, et al. A prospective study of body mass, height, and smoking on the risk of colorectal cancer in women. *Cancer Causes Contr* 1991;2:117–24.

26. Kristal BS, Yu BP. Aging and its modulation by dietary restriction. In: Yu BP, ed. *Modulation of aging processes by dietary restriction.* London: CRC Press, 1994:1–36.

27. Stocks P. Breast cancer anomalies. *Br J Cancer* 1970;24:633–643. Outwater JL, Nicholson A, Barnard N. Dairy products and breast cancer: the IGF-1, estrogen and bGH hypothesis. *Medical Hypotheses* 1997;48:453–461.

28. De Leon DD, Wilson DM, Powers M, Rosenfeld RG. Effects of insulin-like growth factors (IGFs) and IGF receptor antibodies on the proliferation of human breast cancer cells. *Growth Factors* 1992;6:326–336. Outwater JL, Nicolson A, Barnard N. Dairy products and breast cancer: the IGF-1, estrogen, and bGH hypothesis. *Medical Hypotheses* 1997;48:453–461.

29. Albanes D, Jones DY, Schatzkin A, et al. Adult stature and risk of cancer. *Cancer Res* 1988;48:1658–62. Thorling EB. Obesity, fat intake, energy balance, exercise and cancer risk, A review. *Nutrition Res* 1996;16:315–68. Baanders AN, de Waard E. Breast cancer in Europe: the importance of factors operating at an early age. *Eur J Cancer Prev* 1993;2:1–89. Wang DY, Se Stavola BL, Allen DS, et al. Breast cancer risk is positively associated with height. *Breast Cancer Res Treat* 1997;43(2):123–8.

30. Baron S. Niosh study refutes myth of early death. *The New Audible* (National Football League Player Association Newsletter)1994;17(1):1–2.

31. Heitmann BL, Erikson H, Ellsinger BM, et al. Mortality associated with body fat, fat-free mass and body mass index among 60-year-old Swedish men—a 22-year follow-up. The study of men born in 1913. *Int J Obes Relat Metab Disord* 2000;17(1):33–37.

32. Engeland A, Tretle S, Bjorge T. Height, body mass index, and ovarian cancer: a follow-up of 1.1 million Norwegian women. *J Natl Cancer Inst* 2003;95(16):1244–1248.

33. Roth GS, Ingram DK, Black A, Lane MA. Effects of reduced energy intake on the biology of aging; the primate model. *Eur J Clin Nutr* 2000;54(S3):S15–S20.

34. WHO-Global cancer rates could increase by 50% to 15 million by 2020. April 23, 2003 press release. View at www.who.int/mediacentre/releases/2003/pr27/en

35. Carroll KK. Experimental evidence of dietary factors and hormone dependent cancers. *Cancer Res* 1975;35:3374.

36. McPherson K, Steel CM, Dixon JM. ABC of Breast Disease, Breast cancer—epidemiology, risk factors, and genetics. *BMJ* 2000;321:624–628. WHO mortality database at WHO Statistical Information System (WHOSIS).

37. Sullivan MG. More fiber, less fat may reduce breast cancer risk. *Family Practice News* 2003; Jan 11:30.

38. Hilakivi-Clarke E, Cho S, deAssis S, et al. Maternal and prepubertal diet, mammary development and breast cancer risk *J Nutr* 2001;131:154S–157S.

39. UK Department of Health, Working Group on Diet and Cancer of the Committee

on Medical Aspects of Food and Nutrition Policy. *Nutritional aspects of the development of cancer*. London: Her Majesty's Stationary Office, 1998.

40. Pike MC, Henderson BE, Casagrande JT. IN: Pike MC, Siiteri PK, Welsh CN, eds. *Hormones and cancer*. New York, Banbury Reports, Cold Springs Harbor Laboratory 3, 1981.

41. Swerdlow AJ, De Stavola BL, Floderus B, et al. Risk factors for breast cancer at young ages in twins: an international population-based study. *J Natl Cancer Inst* 2002;94(16):1238–1246.

42. Hamilton AS, Mack TM. Puberty and Genetic Susceptibility to Breast Cancer in a Case-Control Study in Twins 2003;348(23):2313–2322.

43. Neergaard L. Early signs of puberty evident. The Associated Press, Washington, D.C. 2/12/01.

44. Berkey CS, Gardner JD, Frazier L, Colditz GA. Relation of childhood diet and body size of menarche and adolescent growth in girls. *Am J Epidemiol* 2000;152(5): 446–452.

45. Baanders AN, de Waard EL. Breast cancer in Europe and factors operating at an early age. *Eur J Cancer Prev* 1993;2:1–89.

46. Yu H, Shu XO, Shi R, et al. Plasma sex steroid hormones and breast cancer risk in Chinese women. *Int J Cancer* 2003;105(1):92–97. Lippman ME, Krueger KA, Eckert S, et al. Indicators of lifetime estrogen exposure: effect on breast cancer incidence and interaction with raloxifene therapy in the multiple outcomes of raloxifene evaluation study participants. *J Clin Oncol* 2001;19(12):3111–3116.

47. Dorgan JF, Hunsberger SA, McMahon RP, et al. Diet and sex hormones in girls: findings from a randomized controlled clinical trial. *J Natl Cancer Inst* 2003;95(2): 132–141.

48. Cho E, Spiegelman D, Hunter DJ, et al. Premenopausal fat intake and risk of breast cancer. *J Natl Cancer Inst* (United States), Jul 16 2003, 95(14):1079–1085.

49. Wolfe JN. Breast parenchymal patterns and their changes with age. *Radiology* 1976;121(2 Pt.1):5454–5552.

50. Llobet JM, Domingo JL, Bocio A, et al. Human exposure to dioxins through the diet in Catalonia, Spain: carcinogenic and non-carcinogenic risk. *Chemosphere* 2003;50(9): 1193–1200.

51. Jensen E, Bolger M. Exposure Assessment of dioxins/furans consumed in dairy foods and fish. *Food Addit Contam* 2001;18(5):395–403.

52. Damastra T. Potential effects of certain persistant organic pollutants and endocrine disrupting chemicals on the health of children. *J Toxicol Clin Toxicol* 2002;40(4):457–465.

53. Janssens J. How nutrition during the first few decades of life affects breast cancer risk implications for research and dietary guidelines for children. *Nutrition Today* Sept 1999.

54. American Cancer Society. Cancer facts & figures 2002. Available at http://www.cancer.org/downloads/STT/CancerFacts&Figures2002TM.pdf.

55. La Vecchia C, Negri E, Parazzini F, et al. Height and cancer risk in a network of case-controlled studies from Northern Italy. *Int J Cancer* 1990;45:275–279.

56. Brunk D. Large study links height to higher risk of prostate cancer. *Family Practice News,* May 1 2003;34.

57. Haenzel W, Kurihara M. Studies of Japanese migrants. Mortality from cancer and other diseases among Japanese in the United States. *J Natl Cancer Inst* 1968;40:43–68.

58. Anderson SO, Baron J, Wolk A, et al. Early life risk factors for prostate cancer: a population-based case-control study in Sweden. *Cancer Epidemiology, Biomarkers & Prevention* 1995;4:187–192.

59. Giovannucci E, Rimm EB, Stampfer MJ, et al. Height, body weight, and risk of prostate cancer. *Cancer Epidemiology, Biomarkers & Prevention* 1997;6:557–563.

60. Sakr WA, Hass GP, Cassin BF, et al. The frequency of carcinoma and intraepithelial neoplasia of the prostate in young male patients. *J Urol* 1993;150:379–385. Cheville JC, Bostwick DG. Postatrophic hyperplasia of the prostate. A Histological mimic of prostatic adenocarcinoma. *Am J Surg Pathol* 1995;19:1068–1076.

61. Ganmaa D, Li XM, Wang J, et al. Incidence and mortality of testicular and prostatic cancers in relation to world dietary practices. *Int J Cancer* 2002;98(2):262–267.

62. Leiss JK, Savitz DA. Home pesticide use and childhood cancer: a case controlled study. *Am J Public Health* 1995;85(2):249–252. Infante-Rivard C, Labuda D, Krajinovic M, Sinnett D. Risk of childhood leukemia associated with exposure to pesticides and with gene polymorphisms. *Epidemiology* 1999;10(5):481–487. Daniels JL, Olshan AF, Savitz DA. Pesticides and childhood cancers. *Environ Health Perspect* 1997;105(10): 1068–1077. Zahm SH, Ward MH. Pesticides and childhood cancer. *Environ Health Perspect* 1998;106(Suppl3):893–908.

63. Bruckner JV. Differences in sensitivity of children and adults to chemical toxicity: the NAS panel report. *Regul Toxicol Pharmacol* 2000;31(3):280–282. Lefferts LY. Pesticide residues variability and acute dietary assessment: a consumer perspective. *Food Addit Contam* 2000;17(7):511–517.

64. Sanderson WT, Talaska G, Zaebst D, et al. Pesticide prioritization for a brain cancer case-control study. *Environ Res* 1997;74(2):133–144. Zahm SH, Blair A. Cancer among migrant and seasonal farmworkers: an epidemiologic review and research agenda. *Am J Ind Med* 1993;24(6):753–766.

65. Wolff MS, Toniolo PG, Lee EW, et al. Blood levels of organochlorine residues and risk of breast cancer. *J Natl Cancer Inst* 1993;85(8):648–652.

66. Reynolds JD. International pesticide trade: is there any hope for the effective regulation of controlled substances? *Journal of Land Use & Environmental Law,* 1997;13(1). Whitford F, Mason L, Winter C. Pesticides and food safety. Purdue University Cooperative Extension Service, PPP-22, Jan. 17, 2005.

67. Worthington V. Nutritional quality of organic versus conventional fruits, vegetables, and grains. *J Alt Compl Med* 2001;7(2):161–173.

68. Grinder-Pedersen L, Rasmussen SE, Bugel S, et al. Effect of diets based on foods from conventional versus organic production on intake and excretion of flavonoids and markers of antioxidative defense in humans. *J Agric Food Chem* 2003;51(19): 5671–5676.

69. Vikari JS, Raitakari OT, Simell O. Nutritional influences on lipids and future atherosclerosis beginning prenatally and during childhood. *Curr Opin Lipidol* 2002;13(1): 11–18.

70. Eriksson JG, Forsen T, Tuomilehto J, et al. Catch-up growth in childhood and death from coronary heart disease: longitudinal study. *BMJ* 1999;318(7181):427–431.

71. Berenson GS, Srinivasan SR, Nicklas TA. Atherosclerosis: a nutritional disease of childhood. Bogalusa Heart Study. *Am J Cardiol* 1998;82(10B):22T–29T. Berenson GS. Childhood risk factors predict adult risk associated with subclinical cardiovascular disease. The Bolgulusa Heart Study. *Am J Cardiol* 2002;90(10C):3L–7L. Vos LE, Orien A, Uiterwaal C, et al. Adolescent blood pressure and blood pressure tracking into young adulthood are related to subclinical atherosclerosis: the atherosclerosis risk in young adults (ARYA) study. *Am J Hypertens* 2003 16(7):549–555.

72. Ludwig DS, Pereira MA, Kroenke CH, et al. Dietary fiber, weight gain, and cardiovascular disease risk factors in young adults. *JAMA* 1999;282(16):1539–1546.

73. My notes from his lecture at symposium sponsored by Intermountain Pediatric Society 1986.

74. Sarasua S, Savitz DA. Cured and broiled meat consumption in relation to childhood cancer: Denver Colorado. *Cancer Causes Control* 1994;5(2):141–148.

75. Clemmesen J. Is smoking in pregnancy a cause of testicular cancer? *Ugesr Laeger* 1997;159(46):6815–6819.

4. FEEDING YOUR FAMILY FOR SUPERIOR HEALTH

1. Bracken MB, Triche EW, Belanger K, et al. Association of maternal caffeine consumption with decrements in fetal growth. *Am J Epidemiol* 2003;157(5):456–466. Vik T, Bakketeig LS, Trygg KU, et al. High caffeine consumption in the third trimester of pregnancy: gender-specific effects on fetal growth. *Paediatr Perinat Epidemiol* 2003;17(4):324–331. Rasch V. Cigarette, alcohol, and caffeine consumption: risk factors for spontaneous abortion. *Acta Obstet Gynecol Scand* 2003;82(2):182–188.

2. Udall JN, Suskind RM. Cow's milk versus formula in older infants: consequences for human nutrition. *Acta Paediatr Suppl* 1999;88(430):61–67.

3. Briefel RR, Reidy K, Karwe V, Devaney B. Feeding infants and toddlers study: Improvements needed in meeting infant feeding recommendations. *J Am Diet Assoc* 2004;104(1 Suppl):s31–s37.

4. Mennella JA. Prenatal and postnatal flavor learning by human infants. *Pediatrics* 2001;107(6):E8dd8.

5. Fisher JO, Mitchell DC, Smiciklas-Wright H, Birch LL. Parental influences on young girls' fruit and vegetable, micronutrient, and fat intakes. *J Am Diet Assoc* 2002;102(1):58–64.

6. Hood MY, Moore LL, Sundarajan-Ramamurti A, et al. Parental eating attitudes and the development of obesity in children. The Framingham Children's Study. *Int J Obes Relat Metab* Disord 2000;24(10):1319–1325.

7. Fisher JO, Mitchell DC, Smiciklas-Wright H, Birch LL. Parental influences on young girls' fruit and vegetable, micronutrient, and fat intakes. *J Am Diet Assoc* 2002;102(1):58–64.

8. Birch LL, Fisher JO. Food intake regulation in children. Fat and sugar substitute and intake. *Ann NY Acad Sci* 1997;819:194–220.

9. Stevens VJ, Glasgow RE, Toobert DJ, et al. Randomized trial of a brief dietary intervention to decrease consumption of fat and increase consumption of fruits and vegetables. *Am J Health Promot* 2002;16(3):129–134.

10. Dorgan JF, Hunsberger SA, McMahon RP, et al. Diet and sex hormones in girls: findings from a randomized controlled clinical trial. *J Natl Cancer Inst* 2003;95(2):132–141.

11. Key TJA, Thorogood M, Appleby PN, Burr ML. Dietary habits and mortality in 11,000 vegetarians and health conscious people: results of a 17 year follow up. *British Medical Journal* 1996;313:775–779.

12. Nelson NJ. Is chemoprevention research overrated or underfunded? *Primary Care & Cancer* 1996;16(8):29–30.

13. Chang-Claude J, Frentzel-Beyme R. Dietary and lifestyle determinants of mortality among German vegetarians. *International Journal of Epidemiology* 1993;22(2): 228–236. Kahn HA, Phillips RI, Snowdon DA, Choi W. Association between reported diet and all cause mortality: Twenty-one year follow up on 27,530 adult Seventh-Day Adventists. *Am J Epidemiol* 1984;119:775–787. Nestle M. Animal v. plant foods in human diets and health: is the historical record unequivocal? *Proc Nutr Soc* 1999;58(2):211–228.

14. Barnard ND, Nicholson A, Howard JL. The medical costs attributed to meat consumption. *Preventive Medicine* 1995;24:646–655. Segasothy M, Phillips PA. Vegetarian diet: panacea for modern lifestyle disease? *QJM* 1999;92(9):531–544.

15. Gillman MW, Cuples LA, Millen BE, et al. Inverse association of dietry fat with development of ischeimic stroke in men. *JAMA* 1997;278:2145–2150. Iso HM, Stampfer MJ, Manson JE, et al. Prospective study of fat and protein intake and risk of intraparenchymal hemorrhage in women. *Circulation* 2001;103:856. Sasaki S, Zhang XH, Kestleloot H. Dietary sodium, potassium, saturated fat, alcohol and stroke mortality. *Stroke* 1995;26(5):783–789.

16. Tully AM, Roche HM, Doyle R, et al. Low serum cholesterol ester-docosahexaenoic acid levels in Alzheimer's disease: a case-control study. *Br J Nutr* 2003;89(4):483–489. Conquer JA, Tierney MC, Zecevic J, et al. Fatty acid analysis of blood plasma of patients with Alzheimer's disease, other types of dementia and cognitive impairment. *Lipids* 2000;35(12):1305–1312.

17. Ophir O, Peer G, Gilad J, et al. Low blood pressure in vegetarians: the possible role of potassium. *Am J Clin Nutr* 1983;37:755–62. Melby CL, Hyner GC, Zoog B. Blood pressure in vegetarians and non-vegetarians: a cross-sectional analysis. *Nutr Res* 1985;5:1077–82. Melby CL, Goldflies DG, Hyner GC, Lyle RM. Relation between vegetarian/nonvegetarian diets and blood pressure in black and white adults. *Am J Publ Health* 1989;79:1283–8. Rouse IL, Armstrong BK, Beilin LJ, Vandongen R. Blood-pressure-lowering effect of a vegetarian diet: controlled trial in normotensive subjects. *Lancet* 1983;1:5–10. Rouse IL, Belin LJ, Mahoney DP, et al. Nutrient intake, blood pressure, serum and urinary prostaglandins and serum thromboxane B_2 in a controlled trial with a lacto-ovo-vegetarian diet. *J Hypertension* 1986;4:241–50. Margetts BM, Beilin LJ, Armstrong BK, Vandongen R. A randomized controlled trial of a vegetarian diet in the treatment of mild hypertension. *Clin Exp Pharmacol Physiol* 1985;12:263–6. Margetts BM,

Beilin LJ, Vandongen R, Armstrong BK. Vegetarian diet in mild hypertension: a randomised controlled trial. *Br Med J* 1986;293:1468–71. Lindahl O, Lindwall L, Spangberg A, et al. A vegan regimen with reduced medication in the treatment of hypertension. *Br J Nutr* 1984;52:11–20.

18. West RO, Hayes OB. Diet and serum cholesterol levels: a comparison between vegetarians and nonvegetarians in a Seventh-day Adventist group. *Am J Clin Nutr* 1968;21:853–62. Sacks FM, Ornish D, Rosner B, et al. Plasma lipoprotein levels in vegetarians: the effect of ingestion of fats from dairy products. *JAMA* 1985;254:1337–41. Fisher M, Levine PH, Weiner B, et al. The effect of vegetarian diets on plasma lipid and platelet levels. *Arch Inter Med* 1986;146:1193–7. Burslem J, Schonfeld G, Howald M, et al. Plasma apoprotein and lipoprotein lipid levels in vegetarians. *Metabolism* 978;27:711–9. Cooper RS, Goldberg RB, Trevisan M, et al. The selective lowering effect of vegetarianism on low density lipoproteins in a cross-over experiment. *Atherosclerosis* 1982;44:293–305.

19. Chang-Claude J, Frentzel-Beyme R, Eilber U. Mortality pattern of German vegetarians after 11 years of follow-up. *Epidemiology* 1992;3:395–401. Thorogood M, Mann J, Appleby P, McPherson K. Risk of death from cancer and ischaemic heart disease in meat and non-meat eaters. *Brit Med J* 1994;308:1667–70. Block G. Epidemiologic evidence regarding vitamin C and cancer. *Am J Clin Nutr* 1991;54:1310S–4S.

20. Pixley F, Wilson D, McPherson K, Mann J. Effect of vegetarianism on development of gallstones in women. *Br Med J* 1985;291:11–2. Frentzel-Beyme R, Claude J, Eilber U. Mortality among German vegetarians: first results after five years of follow-up. *Nutr Cancer* 1988;11:117–26. Burr ML, Batese J, Fehily AM, Leger AS. Plasma cholesterol and blood pressure in vegetarians. *J Human Nutr* 1981;35:437–41. Rouse IL, Armstrong BK, Beilin LJ, Vandongen R. Vegetarian diet, blood pressure and cardiovascular risk. *Aust NZ J Med* 1984;14:439–43.

21. de Ridder CM, Thijssen JHH, Vant Veer P, et al. Dietary habits, sexual maturation, and plasma hormones in pubertal girls: a longitudinal study. *Am J Clin Nutr* 1991;54:805–13. Beaton GH, Bengoa JM. WHO monograph. 1976;62:500–19.

22. Oakley A, Bendelow G, Barnes J, et al. Health and cancer prevention: knowledge and beliefs of children and young people. *BMJ* 1995;310(6986):1029–1033.

23. McNamara D. Obesity behind rise in incidence of primary hypertension. *Family Practice News* April 1, 2003;45.

24. Johnson JG, Cohen PC, Kasen S, Brook JS. Childhood adversities associated with risk for eating disorders or weight problems during adolescence or early adulthood. *Am J Psychiatry* 2002;159:394–499.

25. Barr SI, Janelle KC, Prior JC. Vegetarian vs nonvegetarian diets, dietary restraint, and subclinical ovulatory disturbances: prospective 6-month study. *Am J Clin Nutr* 1994;60:887–894. Janelle KC, Barr SI. Nutrient intakes and eating behavior scores of vegetarian and nonvegetarian women. *J Am Diet Assoc* 1995;95:180–189.

5. PREPARING HEALTHY FOODS THAT YOUR KIDS WILL LOVE

1. Whiting SJ, Lemke B. Excess retinol intake may explain the high incidence of osteoporosis in northern Europe. *Nutr Rev* 1999;57(6):192–195. Melhus H, Michaelson K, Kindmark A, et al. Excessive dietary intake of vitamin A is associated with reduced bone mineral density and increased risk of hip fracture. *Ann Intern Med* 1998;129(10):770–778.

2. Goodman GE. Prevention of lung cancer. *Current Opinion in Oncology* 1998;10(2):122–126. Kolata G. Studies find beta carotene, taken by millions, can't forestall cancer or heart disease. *New York Times,* Jan 19, 1996. Omenn GS, Goodman GE, Thornquist MD, et al. Effects of a combination of beta carotene and vitamin A on lung cancer and cardiovascular disease. *New England Journal of Medicine* 1996;334(18): 1150–1155. Hennekens CH, Buring JE, Manson JE, et al. Lack of effect of long-term supplementation with beta carotene on the incidence of malignant neoplasms and cardiovascular disease. *New England Journal of Medicine* 1996;334(18):1145–1149. Albanes D, Heinonen OP, Taylor PR, et al. Alpha-tocopherol and beta-carotene supplements and lung cancer incidence in the alpha-tocopherol, beta-carotene cancer prevention study: effects of base-line characteristics and study compliance. *Journal of the National Cancer Institute* 1996;88(21):1560–1570. Rapola JM, Virtamo J, Ripatti S, et al. Randomized trial of alpha-tocopherol and beta-carotene supplements on incidence of major coronary events in men with previous myocardial infarction. *Lancet* 1997;349(9067): 1715–1720.

Index